Welcome to

THE
EVERYTHING
PARENT'S GUIDES

As a parent, you're swamped with conflicting advice and parenting techniques that tell you what is best for your child. THE EVERYTHING® PARENT'S GUIDES get right to the point about specific issues. They give you the most recent, up-to-date information on parenting trends, behavior issues, and health concerns—providing you with a detailed resource to help you ease your parenting anxieties.

THE EVERYTHING® PARENT'S GUIDES are an extension of the bestselling Everything® series in the parenting category. These family-friendly books are designed to be a one-stop guide for parents. If you want authoritative information on specific topics not fully covered in other books, THE EVERYTHING® PARENT'S GUIDES are the perfect resource to ensure that you raise a healthy, confident child.

Visit the entire Everything® series at *www.everything.com*

THE
EVERYTHING®

PARENT'S GUIDE TO
the Overweight Child

Dear Reader:

Being overweight hurts, especially when you're a child. Aside from the physical dangers of long-term weight issues, such as heart disease and Type 2 diabetes, excess weight exposes kids to emotional pain that is hard to fathom unless you've been there. Maybe you have, which is why you've decided to pick up this book.

Parents of overweight kids are often plagued by guilt and powerlessness, the same feelings your child is battling as she tries to cope with her weight issues. Those emotions can swiftly sabotage a fitness plan. Set aside the blame, and realize that both of you—working together—can make changes that will last a lifetime.

As a consumer medical writer, I often hear from parents who are concerned about an overweight child in their life. Some worry about the potential, or the reality, of these children developing Type 2 diabetes or other chronic health conditions. Others are looking for ways to help their child take off excess weight, but they simply don't know how to start. *The Everything® Parent's Guide to the Overweight Child* was written to assist you in your efforts to define and reach fitness goals as a family. Good luck on your journey.

Paula Ford-Martin

THE
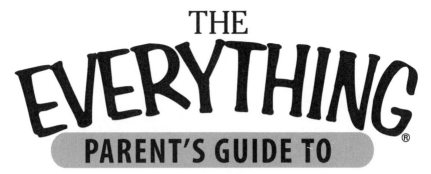
EVERYTHING®

PARENT'S GUIDE TO

THE OVERWEIGHT CHILD

Help your child lose weight, develop healthy
eating habits, and build self-confidence

Paula Ford-Martin,
with technical review by Vincent Iannelli, M.D.

Adams Media
Avon, Massachusetts

For my dad—whose pride and love is always present.

• • •

Publishing Director: Gary M. Krebs
Managing Editor: Kate McBride
Copy Chief: Laura M. Daly
Acquisitions Editor: Kate Burgo
Development Editor: Karen Johnson Jacot
Production Editors: Jamie Wielgus,
Bridget Brace

Production Director: Susan Beale
Production Manager: Michelle Roy Kelly
Cover Design: Paul Beatrice, Matt LeBlanc
Layout and Graphics: Colleen Cunningham
Rachael Eiben, John Paulhus,
Daria Perreault, Monica Rhines, Erin Ring

• • •

An Everything® Series Book.
Everything® and everything.com® are registered trademarks of F+W Publications, Inc.

Published by Adams Media, an F+W Publications Company
57 Littlefield Street, Avon, MA 02322 U.S.A.
www.adamsmedia.com

ISBN: 1-59337-311-2

Printed in Canada.

J I H G F E D C B A

Library of Congress Cataloging-in-Publication Data
Ford-Martin, Paula.
The everything parent's guide to the overweight child / Paula Ford-
Martin with technical review by Vincent Iannelli.
p.   cm. — (An everything series book)
ISBN 1-59337-311-2
1. Obesity in children--Popular works. I. Iannelli, Vincent. II. Title. III. Series: Everything series.

RJ399.C6F67 2005
618.92'398—dc22

2004026531

All the examples and dialogues used in this book
are fictional, and have been created by the author.

overweight child:

a child weighing above the historical 95th percentile of all other children of the same age, height, and gender.

Acknowledgments

Thanks to Vince Iannelli, M.D., for his careful review and comments (and to his wife, brave soul, for letting him take on yet another project with twin toddlers in the house), and to Kate Burgo for her editorial guidance. I'd also like to express my appreciation to fitness guru Paige Waehner for taking the time to share her expertise, and to Barb Doyen, my agent, who is the best cheerleader and advocate a writer could ask for. Finally, a big thank you to my family for their constant love and support.

• • •

Contents

Introduction

Most parents today know very well that more children than ever are overweight or at risk of becoming overweight. Parents have gotten better at recognizing that their own children are overweight, moving away from the denial that a child is just "big boned" or "a little chubby." They may hear about the problem from a pediatrician or a nurse at school. Many parents avoid talking about it in front of their children in order to keep from hurting the children's feelings.

Increasingly, parents are beginning to understand the risks that being overweight poses to their child's health. Not only are these children likely to stay overweight into adulthood and to develop "adult"-type illnesses, like high blood pressure and heart disease, they are also developing diabetes during their teen years at an increasing rate and are at risk of having low self-esteem.

Unfortunately, there are no easy answers to the current obesity epidemic. There is no miracle pill or diet on the horizon that will help kids lose weight. In fact, it seems like today's kids are bombarded with things that actually discourage them from maintaining a healthy weight. This includes poor food choices at school, a lack of opportunities to be physically active at school and after school, oversized portions, drinking too much soda, and so on.

No matter who or what you want to blame for the obesity epidemic, whether it is the fast-food industry, the increased amount of time children spend watching television and playing video games, or parents who make unhealthy choices for their children, one fact remains: It is time to get back to basics and help our children be healthier. Parents probably already know what basic steps have to be taken, including encouraging a child to eat healthy and be physically active every day.

Of course, when it comes to weight loss, things are never simple. Children struggle just as much, if not more, than adults who are trying to lose weight. Why? Part of the reason is a lack of motivation. It can be hard to go from eating whatever you want and spending all day in front of the television to developing healthier habits.

The other big reason is that not all parents really understand how to make healthy food choices or how to provide their children with a nutritious and healthy diet. It is not as easy as counting calories, banning junk food, and getting kids to eat more vegetables. Since they are still growing, children have special nutritional needs. These may not be met if the child is put on a diet that puts too-strict limits on what he eats.

Especially if they are also overweight, parents may have a hard time helping an overweight child. They may not know where to go for help. Although a trip to the pediatrician can be a good idea, parents are unlikely to get all of the help and advice they need in a quick visit. Unfortunately, few parents live near any kind of specialty center dealing with childhood obesity.

Fortunately, that doesn't mean parents are on their own as they work to help an overweight child. *The Everything® Parent's Guide to the Overweight Child* is a wonderful resource for parents interested in helping a child achieve a healthier weight. From identifying and understanding the problem of obesity, to learning to help a child eat right and figuring out how to motivate kids to be more physically active, this book provides parents with all they need to know to help their child lose weight and be healthier.

CHAPTER 1

Generation O: The Obesity Epidemic

W eight problems are nothing new in America. The trend that developed into today's obesity epidemic started well before your child or teen was even born; it's just in the past few years that community leaders, legislators, and educators are starting to sit up and take notice. Today, more than 9 million U.S. children between the ages of six and nineteen are overweight. How did things get so out of hand? What does being overweight mean for your child's long-term health? Most importantly, how do you as a parent effectively help your child control it?

Overweight in America

Well over half of American adults are overweight—a startling 65.7 percent of those over the age of twenty. Of that number, 30.6 percent are considered obese. In 1980, only 47 percent of adults were considered too heavy. What has happened in the past quarter century to make people pack on the pounds?

The National Health and Nutrition Examination Survey (NHANES), conducted each year by the U.S. Centers for Disease Control, takes a look at the health and dietary habits of Americans. In 1971, the survey found that only 4 percent of children ages six to eleven and 6 percent of those age twelve to nineteen were considered overweight. That number has steadily risen. The most recent NHANES data (2001–2002) reports that 16.5 percent of kids between the ages of six and nineteen are overweight, with another 31.5 percent at risk of becoming overweight.

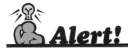

Alert!

Weight is not just a U.S. problem. As documented in its May 2004 report to the World Health Organization, the International Obesity Task Force found that one in ten children around the world—over 155 million—are overweight or obese. The prevalence is rising in both developed and developing countries, and so is the risk of weight-related conditions like Type 2 diabetes and cardiovascular disease.

More men (and boys) than women (and girls) are overweight, in part due to their physical build. (In 2000, 16 percent of boys were overweight versus 14.5 percent of girls.) As a general rule, after puberty, men carry more muscle mass, which is heavier and more metabolically active (that is, burns more calories) than fat tissue, than women do.

Ethnicity can also impact weight. African-American and Hispanic children and teens have a higher rate of weight problems than do Caucasian children. Those trends don't necessarily carry into adulthood; fewer African-American men are overweight than Caucasian men. Yet both male and female Hispanic adults continue to have a higher incidence of weight problems than Caucasian men and women. So do African-American women, who are also at the highest risk for obesity.

Weighing In

Exactly what is "overweight"? The scale can give you a number, but it can't tell you how much of your child's weight is attributable to muscle mass, how her height compares to her weight, or how fat distribution affects her health risks.

There are many tests available for assessing body fat, including skin-fold measurements, bioelectrical impedance, dual energy X-ray absorptiometry (DEXA), and hydrostatic (or underwater) weighing. But the most widely used measurement for determining if your child has a weight problem is the body mass index, or BMI.

Body Mass Index

BMI is a simple calculation based on your child's height and weight (weight in kilograms divided by height in meters, squared). Sometimes additional measurements, such as abdominal circumference, are also taken to assess your child's risk for weight-related medical complications like high cholesterol and insulin resistance. BMI is used to assess overweight and obesity in adults and overweight or risk of becoming overweight in children and adolescents. A child with a BMI between the 85th and 95th percentiles for age and gender is considered to be at risk of becoming overweight, while a BMI at or above the 95th percentile is considered overweight.

 Essential

The bathroom scale doesn't always give the whole picture when you're determining whether your child has a weight problem. Muscle mass is denser, and weighs more, than fatty tissue. If your child is tall and very athletic, it is possible that he could exceed the recommended weight range for his age but still have a healthy body mass index.

The growth charts that your pediatrician uses (discussed in Chapter 3) are based on national data collected by the National Center for Health Statistics from 1963 through 1994. The data has been adjusted to account for an increase in American overweight children and adolescents that began in the 1980s. In actuality, therefore, the percentiles do not reflect exact population references—

for instance, more than 5 percent of American children are considered overweight.

Overweight Versus Obese

In adults, the term "obese" applies to anyone with a BMI in the 97th percentile or higher. However, the U.S. Centers for Disease Control (CDC) recommends that health-care practitioners do not use the term "obese" in reference to children, due to the negative implications of the word. The American Academy of Pediatrics uses the terms "obese" and "overweight" interchangeably in reference to children with a BMI at or over the 95th percentile.

A Heavy Toll

Exactly why is it dangerous for your child to carry too much weight? The most immediate and serious consequence is the possibility of weight-related health problems. Excess fat ultimately requires that your child's heart work harder. Being overweight can also prevent her from getting a good night's sleep, and it puts a strain on her musculoskeletal system. There are psychological consequences as well. Overweight children frequently experience significant emotional turmoil as they attempt to cope with teasing and bullying from insensitive peers. They must also battle doubts about their own self-image and abilities.

Childhood Weight and Health Problems

A host of health problems are associated with excess weight. These include the following:

- **Type 2 diabetes and prediabetes.** Extra weight comes with associated insulin resistance. Though diabetes was once an adult-only disease, prediabetes and Type 2 diabetes are now more common among children and adolescents. In 2004, the CDC predicted that one in three children born in 2000 would develop Type 2 diabetes.
- **Acanthosis nigricans.** This ailment, which involves darkening

and thickening of the folds of the skin (for instance, at the neck and/or armpits), is also associated with insulin resistance.

- **Fatty liver disease.** Also called hepatic steatosis, this condition involves fat accumulation in the liver, and can result in inflammation and scarring (i.e., cirrhosis) of the liver.
- **Hypertension.** Overweight children are more likely to have hypertension, or high blood pressure. Hypertension in youth is a strong predictor of the same condition in adulthood.
- **Hyperlipidemia.** This condition is indicated by a poor cholesterol profile, characterized by elevated LDL (bad) cholesterol and/or triglycerides, and low HDL (good) cholesterol.
- **Cholecystitis.** This condition is indicated by inflammation of the gallbladder. According to the CDC, half of all cases of cholecystitis in adolescents are weight-related.
- **Obstructive sleep apnea.** Breathing is disrupted during sleep due to a blockage of the airway. (See Chapter 15 for more information.)
- **Orthopedic problems**. Overweight children may be placing undue stress on the musculoskeletal system, resulting in knee problems and other orthopedic conditions.
- **Pseudotumor cerebri.** Here, headache and nausea are caused by increased pressure on the brain.
- **Early puberty.** Although this is not always a serious medical problem, overweight girls are more likely to experience early puberty.

Emotional Trauma

It is heartbreaking to watch your child struggle with the self-image issues, depression, and anxiety that often accompany a weight problem. Overweight teens are more likely to be teased than their peers. They're also more likely to have suicidal thoughts. Weight-related teasing can be a major blow to any child's sense of self-esteem, particularly if the taunting is persistent. Kids who are teased about their size report being depressed more often than their thinner peers, and they also perceive themselves as having a poorer quality of life.

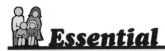
Essential

Help your child develop a strong sense of who she is, and support and nurture her interests, positive friendships, and social pursuits. These steps are the best defense against the confidence-eroding effects of a weight problem. Through both your words and actions, make sure you always reinforce that your child is more than her weight and that you love her at any size.

Why Our Kids Are Getting Fat

A weight problem is usually a matter of losing balance. Weight gain is the result of a simple equation: more calories being eaten than are burned off, through exercise or other physical activity. Children are eating more and moving less. They spend more time sitting still and watching life onscreen than participating in it.

In many cases, they're also following their parents' and peers' lead. When an afternoon with Mom and Dad regularly means sitting and watching a movie and sharing a bucket of buttered popcorn, and when going out with friends means spending the evening munching on fast food and playing video games, it becomes clear that there's a serious disconnect between what people place importance on and what their bodies require for good health.

Learning by Example

Teaching your child good manners, compassion, kindness, and social skills like sharing is probably an everyday priority in your home. It's something you spend as much time on as you do promoting good academic habits. Most parents model these behaviors as much as they can, particularly when a child is very young. But has it been a priority in your household to model regular physical activity and good nutrition?

Kids learn by example, whether it's a good one or a bad one. Even if your child is already a teen, you are his primary role model. When he sees his parents hit the couch after dinner and stay there until bedtime, he assumes that's the norm. Why not spend Saturday afternoon with a bag of chips and a video game and Sunday with donuts and the newspaper if that's the way Dad spends his weekend?

That's why you can't expect your child's fitness plan to be a solitary venture. Every member of the family—parents, siblings, and even the dog (if he'll acquiesce)—must educate themselves on healthy habits and work together towards nutrition and exercise goals. The good news is that it's never too late to get started. Chapter 4 has more information on getting your family with the program.

Cybersloth

Clearly, today's child spends a lot more time on sedentary pursuits like PlayStation and instant messaging than their parents did when they were children. Of all kids between the ages of two and seventeen, 92 percent play video games, and two out of three have some kind of home gaming system. Eighty-three percent of all American households with children have a home computer, and 78 percent of those are online. All told, kids spend an average of six and a half hours *each day* in front of a media screen of some sort (such as the television, movies, computer, or video game). Physical activity is at an all-time low among children and adolescents; over a third of high school students don't get any daily vigorous exercise—that is, exercise that causes perspiration, elevated heart rate, and hard breathing.

Teens are high-volume consumers of media, and because of their growing autonomy and disposable income, they represent a particularly attractive demographic for advertisers to target. Today's teen spends about forty-five minutes a day online (more if he's between the ages of fifteen and seventeen), plays video games for fifty-five minutes daily, and watches television for just over three hours per day. And the trend isn't limited just to "tweens" and teens. A Kaiser Family Foundation study found that a third of all children aged six and younger had their own televisions in their bedrooms, and 27 percent have a VCR or DVD player. On any given day, two-thirds of American children aged six or younger spend an average of two hours watching "screen" media (television, video games, movies, or computer).

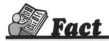 **Fact**

The 1980s was the decade that marked the beginning of the increase in childhood weight gain in America, a trend that would continue for the next quarter century. It is also the decade in which the personal computer and gaming revolution really started to take off, with more reliable, lower-priced systems and better game graphics. (Pac-Man hit the arcades in 1980, and the Commodore 64 debuted in 1982.) Today's kids have a lot more bandwidth to play with than ColecoVision ever offered, which means more time spent on the couch.

There's nothing wrong with your child engaging in age-appropriate television and movie viewing, gaming, and online activities, as long as it's for a reasonable amount of time and she is still getting the physical activity she requires. The growing number of media options and greater access to them can make this a parental challenge, but the goal is an achievable one. Chapter 10 has information on how much exercise your child should be getting.

Genetics and Heredity

Overweight parents are statistically more likely to have overweight children, though whether that's due to nature, nurture, or (most likely) a combination of the two remains to be seen.

Your size and shape, along with that of your child's other parent, is hard-coded into his genetic blueprint. If you are shaped like an eggplant and your husband like a tomato, it's doubtful your child will turn out to be a celery stalk. While inheriting a certain body frame type may be inevitable, your child can influence how he pads it through proper nutrition and regular exercise.

Researchers have theorized that an inherited genetic trait known as the "thrifty genotype" may be responsible for the growing problem of obesity worldwide. Your ancestors may have had specific genetic programming that slowed their metabolism to store body fat when food was plentiful (hence the term "thrifty"). In times of famine, that stored fat became available and allowed them to survive. Today, that same genotype can cause weight to balloon in people living a Westernized lifestyle characterized by high calories and low physical exertion.

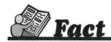**Fact**

Specific "thrifty" genetic tendencies are found in several tribes of native North Americans, including the Pima Indians of Arizona and the Ojibwa-Cree of Manitoba, Ontario. An estimated 70 percent of the Pima are considered clinically obese, and the tribe also has a high incidence of Type 2 diabetes.

Medical Conditions

There are several genetic disorders that can impact body weight, though most of them are rare. These include Bardet-Biedl syndrome and Prader-Willi syndrome, a condition that affects the appetite-regulating function of the hypothalamus, resulting in uncontrolled eating. Endocrine disorders (that is, conditions characterized by hormonal imbalances) and autoimmune diseases that often have weight gain as a symptom include Cushing's disease, polycystic ovary syndrome (PCOS), hypothyroidism, and Hashimoto's thyroiditis.

This list is not all-inclusive. You should talk to your child's pediatrician if you suspect your child's weight may be related to a medical condition. A visit to a qualified health-care professional is an essential part of starting your child on a fitness program, regardless of the cause of her weight problem. Chapter 3 has more information on working with a health-care team.

Food in America

From the time they are old enough to watch a television set or even to visit the grocery store with mom or dad, kids are inundated with advertising for character-shaped, marshmallow-fortified, frosting-crusted cereals and other fat- and sugar-filled junk foods. The food-processing industry spends billions each year on targeting its advertising toward children and teens. Few of those commercials are for fruits and vegetables.

The World Health Organization (WHO) has cited the increased consumption of processed foods heavy in the three S's—saturated fat, sodium, and sugar—as one of the factors behind growing obesity and weight-related health conditions worldwide. In its draft guideline, "WHO Global Strategy on Diet, Physical Activity and Health," the organization has encouraged both government and the food industry to take steps toward reducing salt, fat, and sugar in processed food.

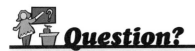

Question?

Has packaged food really gotten that much more fattening in the past few years?

A weight problem is almost always attributable to more than just a single factor. However, a study published in the *American Journal of Clinical Nutrition* found that the use of high-fructose corn syrup as a food ingredient and additive grew by 1000 percent between 1970 and 1990, an increase that researchers found paralleled the rising rates of overweight and obesity in the United States.

Stretching the Food Chain Beyond Recognition

"Creative" kid food concepts have become all the rage, like green ketchup and neon shades of yogurt. But when your child eats these products, he is also getting added chemicals and colorings with his meals. Preservatives, sugar, and fat added during processing can leave even wholesome-sounding foods like fruit juice or muffins barren of nutrients. As a general rule, the further food gets from its original and organic state, and the longer it takes to get from the source to you, the fewer nutrients you (and your child) will get out of it. The best idea is to make whole foods—like fresh veggies, fruits, and whole-grain breads—a primary part of your child's diet.

Misleading Labels

As you start planning a more nutritious lifestyle for your child and your family, you start down the road to being an informed consumer. Become a label reader, and be on the lookout for red-flag ingredients like hydrogenated and partially hydrogenated oils (which signal trans fats, as described in Chapter 6). Look past the advertising slogans that claim foods are low-fat, reduced-calorie, and "light" (or "lite"), and analyze the nutrition facts label. The U.S. Food and Drug Administration (FDA) regulates the way these and other food-related statements may be used, but the FDA's definition of "light," for instance, may be different from yours. To meet FDA guidelines, the food is simply required to contain 50 percent or less of the specific nutrient (such as calories, fat, sodium, cholesterol), depending on the claim, as compared to a "reference food value." While a light cheesecake may be light in comparison to the "real deal," it can still contain substantial amounts of fat and calories.

Bigger Is Better Mentality

Americans are bargain-hunters at heart—hence the American love affair with all-you-can-eat buffets, huge restaurant portions, buy-one-get-one-free pizza deals, and the bottomless beverage. Although these "values" might help you save your pocket change, they cost you plenty more in terms of your good health. All that extra food means American adults and children alike are eating way too many calories. Since we're also less physically active, weight gain is the inevitable result. The added saturated fat in many of the most popular "value-added size" foods, like French fries and movie popcorn, is also clogging arteries and promoting heart disease.

The food-service industry seems to be waking up to the health crisis, at least for now. In 2004, McDonald's announced plans to drop super-sized fries from their menu after considerable bad press about the chain's possible role in America's obesity epidemic. Consumers are becoming more nutrition-savvy and are considering the fiber, fat, and carbohydrate content in many meals before buying. As a result, some chains have added heart-healthy and low-carb options to their menus. More importantly, some are offering their patrons nutritional analyses of menu items so parents can see exactly what their kids are eating.

Of course, unhealthy practices of food manufacturers and restaurants are only one part of the problem. Kids and their parents need to recognize why they make the food choices they do. Kids also have to figure out what triggers overeating behaviors before they can institute long-lasting nutritional lifestyle changes.

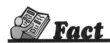 **Fact**

In 1999, Americans consumed 22 million tons of sugar and other sweeteners (such as maple syrup, corn syrup, and honey), according to the U.S. Department of Agriculture. That's 158 pounds per person, or 227,520 calories from sweets a year. Along with all that sugar, U.S. consumers also ate an average of 68.5 pounds of fats and oils in food products.

Overweight Kids Become Overweight Adults

Obesity is often a family disease. Overweight kids grow up to be overweight parents, who in turn have overweight kids themselves. Children of obese parents are more than twice as likely to become obese when they reach adulthood. For overweight kids whose parents are not overweight, the longer the weight stays on, the more likely it is to follow them into adulthood. Children under three who are overweight do not run any additional risk of becoming an overweight adult. But a child who is still overweight after the age of six is 50 percent more likely to become an obese adult than nonoverweight children of the same age.

Clinical studies have demonstrated that the family approach works over the long haul. A ten-year follow-up study at the University of Pittsburgh found that when both parent and child were targeted for weight-loss interventions, the child was more likely to keep off the weight than children in a control group, where the child alone was targeted.

You have the power to break the cycle. Make a commitment to institute new traditions in your family, including fun and challenging exercise, nutritious meals, and open and honest communication with your child. You'll not only help your child achieve her fitness goals and establish good habits that will follow her into adulthood, but you'll emerge with a stronger and healthier family.

CHAPTER 2

Feeding Frenzy: Why Kids Eat Inappropriately

C hildren are extremely impressionable. Their adult role models, peers, and the media messages they encounter all play a part in developing their nutrition and fitness behaviors. These cultural influences can program them to ignore the normal physiological cues that regulate food intake. The good news is that children are also highly adaptable. Once you identify and understand the forces that can work against healthy eating, you can teach them how to cope—and eat—appropriately.

Learned Behaviors

Kids don't start out life gorging on junk food or ignoring hunger and satiety cues. Like every other behavior in life, kids' nutrition and eating patterns are shaped by their culture, role models, and environment. Learning about those influences and how they affect your child's perception of food is important in building new and healthier habits.

Parental Guidance

Children who see Mom trying to lose weight on a steady diet of protein shakes or who witness Dad eating an entire pepperoni pizza as he watches a football game are getting the signal that eating healthy is not a priority for the family. You simply can't expect your children to eat nutritiously if you aren't setting a good example for them to follow. If you aren't doing so already, start to model the healthy eating behaviors you want your child to adapt. Play by the same rules as well. Parents who forbid eating in front of the television but then park themselves in front of their favorite primetime show with a snack tray are telling their kids that the rules they expect them to follow aren't important enough to be observed by all.

Media Messages

From television and movies to magazines and even food packaging, the media feeds children a steady diet of information on food, weight, and culture that is often contradictory. Commercials and advertising bombard children daily, pushing nutrient-barren snacks and implying that social status is somehow tied to the sugary beverage you drink. At the same time, the message is commonplace in films and television shows that fat kids are funny and lacking in willpower while thin equals beauty and popularity. Kids are set up for failure if they buy into the product push and also invest themselves in the media image of the overweight child.

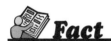 *Fact*

In early 2004, an American Psychological Association (APA) task force (on advertising and children) issued a report calling for restrictions in commercials for children aged eight and younger. Children in this age group believe commercials are completely factual and don't understand the concept of persuasive intent. The APA task force cited the prominence of youth-targeted junk-food commercials as one reason that an eight-and-under ban should be put into place.

According to the Kaiser Family Foundation, the average American child sees more than 40,000 television commercials a year, and the majority of those are marketing food. By acting as gatekeepers, parents can control some of a child's exposure to the more negative messages. But as your children grow older, you need to ensure they have been taught to view commercial and cultural media messages with a critical eye. That includes teaching them healthy eating habits, but it's also important to remind them frequently from an early age that the only purpose of a television commercial is to sell a product.

It can also be helpful to point out commercials that are flat out wrong or that misrepresent a product. It is definitely a disappointing experience for a child to discover that a toy is nowhere near as large as the picture on the box, or that a doll breaks when you try to play with it the way the little girl did on television. However, these are also excellent learning opportunities to show children that advertising isn't always accurate or in their best interests.

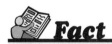 **Fact**

Packaged foods marketed on the basis of their entertainment value, such as jellied fruit-like snacks in character shapes, color-changing beverages and condiments, and cereals with surprises inside, also drive home the message that food is for fun, not for fuel.

Food As Love

Food has a rich and long history of being used as a symbol of love, a tradition that remains with our society today. We give chocolates for Valentine's Day, bring an apple to a favored teacher, and bake a favorite dessert for a visiting friend or family member. But when food starts to become a tangible substitute for healthier displays of affection, communication, and emotional comfort, the stage is set for lifelong eating problems.

Using Food As a Reward or Band-Aid

Your son gets straight A's on his report card. How do you react?

(a) Tell him how proud you are of him and discuss an appropriate reward for his hard work.
(b) Slap him on the back, and say "How about A-pluses next time?"
(c) Take him out for a six-scoop hot fudge sundae with all the trimmings.

If answer "c," with its gift of food, is the first thing that pops into your head when your child reaches a goal or earns a major achievement, it's time to start reevaluating your reward system. Using food as a consistent way to express your pride teaches a child that offering food is your way of showing love. The message that sweets and treats are the most appropriate way of expressing your love is one that can stick with her into adulthood. It's a behavior that can create unhealthy eating patterns that span generations.

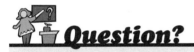 *Question?*

We always take the family out to dinner to celebrate great report cards and other achievements. Is that wrong?
No, not at all. A family celebration is a great way to commemorate your child's accomplishment, and a visit to a restaurant can be a fun time for all. Just make sure that the celebration is focused on your child, that the menu offers plenty of healthy food choices, and that the meal is more about having a good time together as a family than gorging on the dessert tray.

Another common and unhealthy use of food is as a comforting mechanism. The promise of an ice cream cone is a convenient and effective distraction for a child who has just fallen off her bike and banged up her knee, but it also reinforces the concept of food as a panacea for problems. Better would be a hug, kiss, and maybe some of Mom's extra-special bandages.

Sending the Wrong Message

Expressing and experiencing emotions is a healthy and natural process. Sometimes adults forget that, and they offer food to stop tears or get a child's mind off his troubles. While this strategy may be successful when it comes to making the hurt of a skinned knee go away, it certainly won't solve deeper emotional or social problems. If food becomes associated with emotional comfort, it can prevent your child from fully exploring and discussing his feelings with you. Instead of developing the coping and problem-solving skills he needs to become a happy and successful member of society, he learns to run to the refrigerator every time difficulties arise in his life.

No parent wants to see a child in pain, and it's easy to see how parents can fall into the food trap. A special treat makes a toddler stop crying instantly, and a light bulb goes on in the parent's head that says, "Hey—that worked fast!" Ten years later, Mom and Dad are still using the same offer of a treat to help their adolescent child feel better about an argument with a friend or a poor test score. If you recognize yourself in that example, the good news is that it isn't too late to change your approach. You can put food back into perspective and guide your child towards healthier avenues of problem-solving.

Eating Away from Home

Changing meal and eating habits at home is only half the battle in the fight for good nutrition. From school lunches to Saturdays at the mall with friends, your child will be eating more snacks and meals without adult or at least parental supervision as she grows older. If you instill good eating habits in your child at home, she will have the skills to make appropriate food choices most of the time when she's on her own. But even with the knowledge you give them, there are many potential pitfalls awaiting kids when they eat away from home.

Portion Problems

Getting more for your money is one of the concepts that drives American business and culture. Bigger is typically perceived as better, especially when it comes to food. So it's really no surprise that the portions dished out in restaurants today are often many times larger than what one person needs.

A 2003 study by the Child Nutrition Research Center at Baylor University found that on average, preschool-aged kids who were served double-size portions of macaroni and cheese for lunch consumed 25 percent more food, 15 percent more calories, and took bigger bites, regardless of their level of hunger. However, when those same children were allowed to dish out their own meals, they ate age-appropriate portions, indicating that if left to their own devices and allowed to serve themselves, most kids will self-regulate the amounts of food they eat.

 Essential

Don't forget that children don't need adult-sized portions. Allowing your children to dish up their own servings at home can discourage overeating. If they have a tendency to pile too much on their plates, serve meals family-style at the table. Encourage them to take small portions with the assurance that they can dish out more if they're still hungry after their first serving.

So how do you avoid the portion problem away from home? If you're with your child, you can suggest splitting dishes with other diners in your group as you order. There's also the old standby—the doggy bag. If your child is eating out without you, remind him that he should feel free to take half his meal home if it's too much to eat at once.

Beyond quantity, there's also the issue of the quality when it comes to restaurant offerings. While many restaurants have added healthier fare to their menus for weight- and nutrition-conscious adults, standard children's menus continue to lag far behind in nutritional value. Kid cuisine staples include deep-fried, fat-laden, and high-calorie items like cheeseburgers, fries, tater tots, chicken fingers, sodas, and hot fudge sundaes. In some cases, your kids may be better off ordering from the adult menu, so encourage that when no healthier child options are available.

Fast-Food Focus

Another place where super-sizing has reached a critical level is at your favorite fast-food restaurant. Free toys, fries, and fancy playgrounds have made the local burger place a favorite stop for kids. The occasional fast-food lunch may be inevitable, but if you're swinging into the drive-through several times a week, chances are good that your kids are getting too many calorie- and fat-packed meals with few nutrients. If your lifestyle demands food that is quick and easy, there are other options for meals. See Chapter 9 for more information on fast and fit food choices.

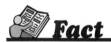 *Fact*

A study of over 6,000 children between the ages of four and nineteen that was published in the journal *Pediatrics* found that on any given day, 30 percent of the study subjects ate fast food. On the whole, frequent fast-food eaters consumed more calories and sugar and less fiber and fruits and (nonstarchy) veggies.

The School Cafeteria

Many parents rely on the school cafeteria. It's the one place a child should be able to count on getting a nutritious, well-balanced meal each day. Unfortunately, this assumption may not hold true in many cases. The National School Lunch Program, which provides federal subsidies to schools for meal programs, relies heavily on dairy and meat commodities. Nutritional analysis of school lunch meals served is based on a weekly menu average, which means that the total and saturated fat content in some individual school lunches can exceed the daily recommended amount for your child. In addition, in some high schools and middle schools, à la carte items are offered that may make the nutritional landscape even bleaker. French fries, brownies, fried cheese, packaged chips and snacks, and other less-than-ideal choices are often available for purchase in addition to, or instead of, the regular school lunch menu. Take a close look at your child's monthly school lunch menu and the à la carte offerings. In some cases, or at least on some days, it may make more sense to send your child to school with a bag lunch. See Chapter 19 for more information on improving school food options.

Ignoring Hunger and Satiety Cues

In an ideal world, kids (and adults) would eat only when hungry and then only enough until they feel full. Unfortunately, kids often eat because the food simply looks too good to pass up, or out of habit because it's time to eat, or simply because they're bored. Sometimes, they'll keep eating until they're well past full because they've gone on autopilot with their eating and are focusing on other things.

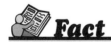 **Fact**

In the Baylor University study of preschoolers and portion size, researchers found that kids who reported eating more snack foods when they weren't really hungry were also more likely to overeat when large portions were provided to them. Children with a higher BMI were also more likely to take larger bites.

If you find your child heading to the refrigerator when he's just eaten a good meal, stop and ask him if he's eating because he's hungry or because he's bored. If the answer is the latter, take a time-out, and go and find something to do together. More importantly, talk with him about really asking himself about his own hunger every time he goes into snack-seeking mode. Then sit down and make a list together of all the things he could do to make life more interesting instead of eating for fun. Make it varied—include quiet activities like reading as well as outdoor fun so he'll have choices in any kind of weather at any time of day—and post it on the refrigerator or inside the pantry door. The next time he looks for food out of boredom, the list will hopefully trigger him to assess his actual hunger and motivate him to go do something else for fun if he finds he's eating to kill time.

Mindful Eating

Eating while performing other tasks such as watching television, playing video games, or talking on the phone can short-circuit feelings of satiety. If you're distracted by other things, it's possible to miss that feeling of fullness that tells you your stomach has had enough. This is the same phenomenon that causes you to eat an entire family-sized bucket of buttered popcorn solo while watching a movie. Encourage your children to practice mindful eating. Ask that all meals and snacks be eaten around the kitchen table. Meals and snacks should be eaten with the television off and with the family when possible.

Listening to Your Child's Cues

Through their well-intentioned efforts to make sure children eat well, parents often ignore their children's hunger and satiety cues. If dinner is on the stove and your child says she's hungry for a snack, do you allow her to have a nutritious bite to eat, or does she have to wait until dinner? If she says she's full but has only eaten half her dinner, and hasn't touched her broccoli, do you excuse her from the table or demand she take a bite or two of the veggies? If you insist on judging adequate nutrition by the clock or the quantity of food left on a plate, an you ignore your child when says she's hungry or full, you're reinforcing the idea that her hunger cues are not important. As a result, she may start disregarding them herself.

Food as a Social Occasion

Events where food is the center of attention can promote eating beyond or in the absence of hunger. The most notorious example for adults is probably Thanksgiving, but children face far more frequent occurrences in which food takes center stage. Birthday parties, holiday treats at school, candy from a teacher, pizza parties, team trips to an ice cream parlor—the list goes on and on. When your child is headed off to a social event, make sure he knows it's okay to say no if he isn't hungry. If it fits the occasion, ask the host if you can contribute some snacks. Send along something healthy that he and his friends can munch on, so you'll know he has choices. For more on kids, food, and special occasions, see Chapter 14.

Emotional Eating

Emotional eating can also cause overeating problems for older children. A child who has a fight with a friend or receives a bad report card may turn to a bag of cookies or other comfort foods. He is using food to make him feel better, rather than talking out his feelings with his parents. Part of this may be learned behavior. If parents push treats as a way to distract a young child from problems instead of dealing with them, the child may not develop appropriate coping skills as he matures. Emotional eating isn't just limited to kids, either. If children see the adults around them drowning their sorrows in chocolate, they will assume that eating is an acceptable way to deal with emotional pain.

If you think your child is turning to food instead of dealing with her problems, encourage her to talk to you about what's troubling her. Let her see you discussing problems and points of conflict with your spouse or others, expressing how these issues make you feel and resolving them instead of ignoring them. It may also be beneficial to seek the help of a child or adolescent therapist.

Eating Disorders

If your child exhibits compulsive behaviors and consumes large quantities of food at a single sitting, he may have an eating disorder that requires intervention by a child psychiatrist, psychologist, or therapist. Binge-eating disorder (BED) is most common in overweight kids and adults, although people of a "normal" BMI can also develop the condition. It most frequently strikes in adolescence and early adulthood. BED is also closely associated with depression.

Potential signs your child may be bingeing include the following:

- Frequent and unaccountable disappearance of bags or packages of food
- Signs of depression
- Insistence that the child be left to eat alone
- Apparent remorse, guilt, or embarrassment related to eating behaviors
- Unexplained weight gain

For a child with BED or any other eating disorder, trying to lose weight without first addressing the underlying causes of the problem is a losing game. If you suspect your child is binge eating, take him to a qualified mental health-care professional with experience in treating eating disorders in children. Eating disorders are discussed in more depth in Chapters 12 and 18.

CHAPTER 3

Acceptance and Action: Identifying the Problem

A s a parent, you may tend to see only the best in your child, which means you may not have really come to terms with her weight issues. Perhaps it took your son's pediatrician mentioning that he was a little large for his age, or a friend's gentle hint that your daughter was "a big girl." Or maybe your child came home in tears, the target of some insensitive schoolyard taunt about his size. Now you're seeing the situation for what it is for the first time. Acknowledging the problem is the first step in helping your child; after acceptance, you can take action.

Your Child's Healthy Weight

What should your child weigh? It's important to remember that a child's ideal weight is not merely a number on a chart, but the place where she feels self-confident, healthy, and strong. Your child's doctor can help you determine a weight range that is physically healthy for her age.

There are national averages—known as standardized growth charts—that help your pediatrician determine if your child's specific growth patterns are on track with that of other children of the same age. However, issues such as whether your child was bottle- or breastfed (and how long), born preterm or at was considered very low birth weight (VLBW), and any history of chronic disease or medical problems can all have an impact on your child's growth patterns and how the standardized growth chart applies.

Don't get too focused on a single "magic number" for your child. A wide range of weights may be considered normal for a single age, and that range can change based on the factors already listed above. In some cases, particularly those in which weight increase suddenly outstrips height growth, with no apparent changes in activity level or diet, weight gain may be a simple matter of the body needing to play catch-up.

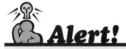

Alert!

Remember that weight isn't an appearance issue as much as it is a health issue. To keep the focus on feeling good, try not to tie weight-loss goals with fitting in to a specific clothing size or being the same weight as a peer.

Charting Your Child's Growth

Your child's doctor has probably told you regularly, probably at each of your child's routine checkups, that your child is in a specific percentile for height and for weight. Like many parents, you probably nodded your head and maybe made a note for your child's baby book or health records. Otherwise, you had no clue exactly what those numbers meant. Or maybe you assumed that a high score meant your child was growing well. Here's your chance to learn what those numbers really mean.

Types of Charts

Your child regularly gets her height and weight measured at the pediatrician's office (and head circumference, at thirty-six months and younger). The doctor plots that information on a graph. The results show your child's growth trends from birth on as well as size in comparison to other children of the same age.

Your doctor has several other national growth charts against which to compare your child, including weight for stature (or height), weight for length, weight for age, stature for age, BMI for age, and head circumference for age (used for charting brain development and detecting potential developmental problems in infants and toddlers). The charts your provider uses will depend upon your child's age and the standard at your doctor's practice.

Essential

The 2000 CDC growth charts are based on survey information compiled from 1963 through 1994. The data has been adjusted to account for the increase in American overweight children and adolescents that began in the 1980s. Therefore, the percentiles do not actually reflect exact population references; for instance, more than 5 percent of today's American children are considered overweight. Still, they are intended to be used as this type of reference guide.

The growth charts that your child's pediatrician uses were developed in 1977 by the U.S. Centers for Disease Control (CDC), using data collected from the National Health Examination Survey (NHES) and the National Health and Nutrition Examination Survey (NHANES). The CDC updated these charts in 2000 to incorporate new data, including revised national statistics for infants and new charts showing the relationship between body mass index and age.

Percentiles

Your child's measurements, as related to those of other children the same age, are expressed in terms of a percentile. Standard CDC growth charts include growth curves from the 5th to the 95th percentile. A set of charts is also available that range from the 3rd to the 97th percentile for use with children who fall above or below the standard charts in weight and/or height. If your son is in the 95th percentile for his weight, it means that he weighs more that ninety-five percent of the statistical sampling of U.S. boys his age. It also means that he weighs less than 5 percent of the boys surveyed. That number by itself doesn't always mean a lot, but when you factor in his body mass index (BMI), which takes his height into account as well, you get a more complete picture.

Body Mass Index

The American Academy of Pediatrics (AAP) recommends that the body mass index (BMI) of children and adolescents be calculated and plotted annually to assess growth patterns. For children and young adults between the ages of two and twenty, the CDC introduced a BMI-for-age chart in 2000. A weight-for-stature chart for the same age group is also available, but the CDC recommends that the former be used because it is more effective as a screening tool.

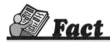 *Fact*

The growth charts used by your child's pediatrician were developed by the National Center for Health Statistics (NCHS) in 1977 using data collected from the National Health and Nutrition Examination Survey (NHANES). In 2000, the CDC updated the charts to incorporate new data, including revised national statistics for infants and new BMI-for-age charts.

Body mass index is a measurement of your child's body weight adjusted for height. It can help your child's doctor screen for weight problems, although it isn't diagnostic in and of itself. This means that further assessment will be required if the BMI indicates your child may have a weight problem. Keep in mind that BMI-for-age charts are not used for children under age two. Studies have found that a high BMI in this age group is not directly associated with either weight-related medical problems or a risk of obesity in adulthood.

To get an accurate BMI reading, your child's physician will first measure height and weight. This information is then plotted on the appropriate CDC height-for-age and weight-for-age growth charts. Once these measurements are taken, BMI can be computed using the following mathematical formula:

BMI = Weight (lb) / Stature (in) / Stature (in) × 703

Note: Stature is equivalent to standing height.

Or, in metric measurements:

BMI = Weight (kg) / Stature (cm) / Stature (cm) × 10,000

Measuring Up

Once your child's BMI is computed, the pediatrician can plot it on the BMI-for-age chart to figure out the BMI percentile—that is, where your child's BMI falls in comparison with other children of the same age. **Table 3-1** shows the percentile indicators for underweight, risk of being overweight, and overweight. Weight-for-length and weight-for-stature indicators are also included for children assessed with those charts.

Table 3-1: Weight Indicators		
Underweight	**Risk of Overweight**	**Overweight**
BMI-for-Age Percentile		
Below the 5th percentile	From the 85th to the 94th percentiles	95th percentile or greater
Weight-for-Length/Stature Percentile		
5th	N/A	95th

Note: Unlike guidelines for adult overweight and obesity, overweight indicators for children are based on percentiles rather than on specific BMI cutoffs. Children are still growing and developing, so it's important to evaluate their size in relationship to their peers rather than the static guidelines used in adulthood.

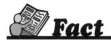 **Fact**

If your child is between the ages of two and five, your provider may use a weight-for-stature chart to plot growth rather than a BMI-for-age chart. The CDC offers these growth charts as a tool for pediatric care providers who are still making the shift to the BMI standard.

Is It Fat or Something Else?

If your child's BMI-for-age falls into a percentile that categorizes him as overweight or places him at risk of becoming overweight, your doctor will need to do some further assessment. It is necessary to determine whether the issue is one of weight or whether there's another underlying problem. Again, BMI is only a screening tool—it's a measure that can't diagnose a weight problem by itself. A child who is involved in athletic activities that build significant muscle mass, such as weight-lifting, may have a high BMI that isn't attributable to excess fat. In addition, children whose parents have large musculo-skeletal frames (tall and broad physiques) may have a higher BMI without being overweight.

To determine whether a weight problem is a possibility, your child's doctor should perform additional assessments, including these:

- **Family history**—Your doctor will ask if there is anything in your family background or medical history to indicate a propensity towards weight problems or weight-related complications, such as Type 2 diabetes and heart disease.
- **Physical examination**—Your child may undergo testing for potential weight-related complications, including cholesterol screening, blood pressure, and blood glucose testing.
- **Skin-fold measurements**—A measurement of skin-fold thickness on the back of the triceps (on the upper arm) of 95 percent or higher is usually considered an indicator of a weight problem.

- **Activity and nutritional assessment**—Your child's doctor may interview you and your child about nutritional intake and exercise habits to determine if there is an imbalance in either that could be causing weight gain.

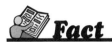 **Fact**

From birth up to age three, your child's growth is plotted on a length-for-age and weight-for-length chart. At these ages, a child's height is measured in a recumbent (lying down) rather than a standing position. Two-year-olds can be plotted on either a weight-for-length or a weight-for-height chart.

Coming to Terms with the Problem

From the moment your child came into this world, you've devoted yourself to protecting her from harm. The discovery that her health and well-being is at risk due to a weight problem can be a painful emotional blow—one that might make you question your self-worth as a parent. You may have faced weight issues yourself, either now or in the past, that have left you with the belief that your child's weight problem was inevitable. You may have been in denial about the problem, calling your child "solid," "husky," "a good eater," or "big-boned" to rationalize a growing weight problem. Or you may just have thought that her size was something she'd grow into with time.

No matter how you arrived at this moment of realization, it's important to forgive yourself and move on. There are almost always a large numbers of reasons behind a child's weight gain, and the finger can't be pointed at any one cause or influence in isolation. For instance, genetic and medical history—two factors over which you have no control—can exert a strong influence on your child's size. Even if you haven't always served the healthiest meals, or you let the kids watch an extra hour of television instead of encouraging active play, it is neither fair nor productive to place the blame solely on yourself as the cause of your child's problems. You've recognized that you need to take action now, and that's what counts.

Banishing Guilt and Blame

Guilt and blame will do nothing positive for you. In fact, these feelings may actually hinder your efforts to help your child get fit. If you place all culpability on yourself, you may go to extremes in trying to fix and control the problem and not allow your child to play an active role in his own health. These negative feelings can also be contagious. Children are more aware of your emotional state that you may realize, and they may feel at fault themselves if they perceive that your anxiety is related to their weight. Guilt and blame can be particularly destructive feelings when experienced by a child and can shatter their sense of self-esteem, which is often fragile anyway. A guilty or ashamed child may also become negatively motivated to lose weight, seeing weight loss as a way of earning your love or making you "feel better." Getting fit needs to be something your child works towards because it's positive and fulfilling for his well-being.

Promise yourself you'll stop feeling bad about where your child's weight is right now. Instead, work to help him develop the tools he needs to make smart choices and move towards his fitness goals.

Taking Action

Your first step in helping your child is to consult with your pediatrician or family doctor about her fitness level. If you're aware your child has a weight problem, you've probably had some discussion with her physician already. However, you may not have gotten the details you need to take effective action against the problem. The next section, "Talking to Your Child's Doctor," provides more detail on consulting with a doctor to develop a safe and effective fitness program for your child.

Discussing fitness with your child, either before or after the doctor's consultation, is also a critical first step. Your child's age will play a large role in how you approach the discussion. Older children may have already come to you with concerns about their weight, while younger kids have a hard time connecting their weight with any unhealthy lifestyle habits. At every age, try not to make comparisons between your child and his peers. Trading weight and height stats with other parents usually only leads to feelings of frustration and inadequacy. It also discounts the fact that each child has a unique set of genetic and environmental influences that contribute to his or her body type.

Talking to Your Child's Doctor

The decision of whether to talk to the doctor in a one-on-one consultation or with your child in attendance will depend on her age and personality. Very young children won't mind being part of the conversation and may benefit from their inclusion. (For younger children in particular, establishing an authority figure aside from the parents can sometimes make it a little easier to enforce new lifestyle changes.) Older kids who are feeling emotionally vulnerable about their weight may feel self-conscious about the discussion, and adolescents may even prefer to meet with the doctor privately.

If your teen meets with the doctor without you, be sure to get a quick recap from the physician on what you need to do to help your child succeed in a fitness plan. You might ask the doctor to take some notes on the main points of the conversation for your child to pass on to you afterwards. That way you aren't encroaching on what your teen feels is private business, but you will still have the information you need to help your child succeed and be able to follow up with the doctor on anything that is unclear to either of you.

Questions to Ask

If your child does attend the session with you, make sure to frame all questions in a positive light. It's also important to include your child in the conversation. A weight-loss plan won't achieve long-term success unless your child is invested in the process and senses that his feelings and participation matter.

Questions to ask your child's physician include the following:

- In what percentile do my child's weight and height fall on the growth charts for his age?
- What is the "ideal" weight range for his age and height, and what do you think his specific goal should be, based on his body type and medical history?
- Should weight maintenance or weight loss be his goal?
- If weight loss is a goal, what amount of weight is realistic and safe for him to lose each week/month?
- Does his current activity level seem appropriate?
- Do you have any sample meal plans and nutritional hand-outs, and can you provide a referral to a registered dietitian for a consultation?

These questions are general guidelines only. If your child has a chronic health condition, food allergies, or other complicating factors in his medical history, you will want to discuss a weight loss plan in the context of those issues.

What to Expect

After you've had an opportunity to discuss your child's current weight and any medical or environmental issues that may be contributing factors, your child's doctor will suggest a plan of either weight maintenance or weight loss, depending on your child's age, BMI, and the presence of any weight-related complications.

In many cases, your child's physician may recommend that your child attempt to keep his weight steady for awhile to let his height catch up with his weight growth. In the case that your child is topping out over the 95th percentile and weight-related health complications are involved, very gradual weight loss may be recommended. Each child's situation is different, and your physician will assess your child individually. Some weight-loss goals will take longer than others to achieve. In all cases, the final target for your child will be to achieve a BMI that is below the 85th percentile for other children of the same age.

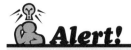
Alert!

According to the CDC, children under the age of seven who need to lower their BMI due to the presence of weight-related complications should generally never lose more than one pound per month. For children seven or older who are overweight and require a weight loss plan, the maximum amount of weight dropped should not exceed one to two pounds per week.

Talking to Your Child

For children who are of preschool or early elementary-school age, any conversations about weight should be very general. Discussion should encouraged the child to enjoy a healthier family lifestyle, choose better foods, get out and about more, and limit couch-potato time. Bringing weight into the conversation is probably not necessary unless your child has brought it up herself. If your child is unselfconscious about her size, making an issue of it can do more harm than good, and could turn the new family focus on fitness into an appearance issue instead of a health issue.

For older children and adolescents, it's quite probable that they are already very aware of their weight problem. Making dramatic changes to meals and suddenly signing the family up for a new gym membership will not pass unnoticed, and your teen may even resent such boldness as a tyrannical attempt to control her lifestyle, no matter how good your intentions. Discuss the issue frankly. Let your child know that fitness is a challenge the entire family will share in and that you are there for support.

Focus on Health Instead of Weight

You've always taught your child that what counts is on the inside and to never judge a book by its cover. These all the other life lessons you've passed along drive home the point that appearance doesn't matter. Yet your child's peers, the media she sees daily, and society all tend to send a much different message—that fat is ugly and thin is in.

It's extremely important that your child understands that you want to help her lose weight to improve her health and her health alone. Now, in all honesty and realism, you of course want to spare your child from the pain that "fat kids" face, such as frequent teasing and being left out of almost anything the other kids decide to do together. It is unfortunately, but older children have probably already been through some degree of emotional pain on account of their size. Your child may even long for the supposed social benefits that weight loss appears to bring. Even so, don't make being "slim and pretty" a goal of this fitness program, or you'll be setting a high value on looks and unintentionally condoning such behavior in the process. Your child needs to know that her parents value her at any size and regardless of her physical appearance.

Finally, the healthy new habits you promote will only take root and become a permanent lifestyle if you stress that they are a means to the long-term benefits of feeling better, having more energy, increasing strength and flexibility, and minimizing weight-related health risks.

Exploring Feelings

As you discuss your child's weight and a plan for promoting a healthier way of living, you may discover a full spectrum of conflicting emotions. He may feel great relief that you are facing the problem together and excitement at the prospect of making real and positive changes. However, he may also be full of less helpful emotions, including at least a few of these:

- **Inward anger**—Your child may blame himself for his weight problem and be full of anger because of it.
- **Outward anger**—Your child may be angry with you for "allowing" the problem to occur, or for pointing out the problem.
- **Helplessness**—Your child may feel a lack of control over his

life and physical fitness level that have left him convinced that he can't make positive changes.

- **Denial**—Your child may refuse to recognize he is overweight, particularly if the problem has gone unmentioned by anyone for quite some time.
- **Resentment**—Your child may state he doesn't want your help or resent your "interference" in his life.
- **Grief**—Your child may feel a sense of loss at the prospect of giving up old, unhealthy habits.

Talk these issues out with your child. Encourage him to be honest about how he is feeling, with the assurance that you won't be angry or disappointed in him no matter what he shares. Everyone needs to vent occasionally, and just letting these feelings out can be beneficial. Often, he just needs to hear your reassurances that you believe in him and are there for him.

 Essential

A child or family therapist may be helpful in some cases, especially if your child seems to harbor strong feelings of anger and resentment that you can't resolve with discussion. Such feelings can hinder a successful weight-loss and fitness plan. They can also place undue stress on your child and family, and sometimes it takes a neutral third party to help break down emotional roadblocks.

Empowering Your Child

Another essential component for positive, healthy change is to allow your child to help plan the road you'll take. Teach him to cook, let him plan your family's weekend fitness time, and let him order for himself when you eat out. Your child needs your guidance, but he also needs to feel some sense of control over his own destiny. Teach him what he needs to know to make smart choices, and then make sure he has plenty of opportunities to make those decisions.

Diet Versus Lifestyle Change

When it comes to helping your child develop healthy habits and reach an improved level of fitness, it's critical to remember that "diet" is a four-letter word. Helping your overweight child is not about cutting out desserts and force-feeding broccoli. It's about embarking on a whole new way of living as a family.

Referring to your new way of eating as a diet doesn't work for several reasons. First of all, a diet implies a short-term plan, one that can be abandoned as soon as a weight goal is reached. Your new way of eating is one that you hope will stay with your child, and your family, for life. The term "diet" also leaves exercise out of the healthy weight equation, although (as we now know) physical activity is an integral part of fitness for children and adults.

When talking about dietary changes with your child, refer to them simply as "healthy eating" or "better food choices." Emphasizing moderation is also key. No food is really inherently bad if consumed in reasonable amounts at appropriate times. A big slab of chocolate fudge cake à la mode for dessert every night of the week isn't the best thing for a child trying to reach a healthier weight level, but the occasional slice of birthday cake is fine. As you're well aware just by virtue of being a parent, slapping a big red "NO" on anything just makes the forbidden seem that much more attractive.

Creating a Supportive Environment

The "Do as I say, not as I do" philosophy is the quickest way to sabotage your child's fitness goals. You need to be a role model in this effort. Think back to the last time you tried to give up a difficult habit or make a major change in your life without adequate support. Perhaps it was giving up cigarettes while your significant other continued to smoke a pack a day, or trying to stick to a strict budget while your best friend dragged you along on her weekly shopping spree. You may or may not have managed to achieve your objective. Either way, it was probably painfully clear that achieving a goal is much harder when those around you are working against you instead of with you.

With that in mind, your whole family—siblings included—should make an effort to make the lifestyle changes that will help your child achieve a healthier weight. Keep cupboards stocked with healthy snacks. Plan active weekend outings, and keep emotionally connected as well. While a trip to the park or a bike ride is a great way to spend active time with your child, quiet times with family spent talking, playing board games, or reading together are just as important to ensuring an emotional connectedness that will help your child feel loved and supported in her efforts. Chapter 4 discusses strategies for putting a stronger family focus on your physical activities and spare time.

Redefining Family Life for Healthier, Happier Kids

Your child didn't gain weight in isolation, and he can't be expected to lose it as a solo act either. Putting together a realistic meal and exercise plan for the entire family to follow is a crucial step in ensuring your child's success. In some cases, this may involve only a few minor lifestyle adjustments. For other families, however, it may mean a complete food and fitness makeover.

A Family Affair

No matter what your family structure, helping your child achieve a healthier weight should involve the entire household. It doesn't matter whether you belong to a traditional nuclear family or single-parent household, whether you are a guardian of your grandchild or parent of one child or a dozen—everyone can benefit from good food, exercise, and the emotional connections that are strengthened when families work towards good health together.

Walking the Walk

When several members of the household have weight issues, the benefits of a family fitness plan are obvious. But sometimes, when parents and siblings happen to be slim, there's a misconception that the only person with "a fitness problem" is the child who is overweight. Take a long, hard look at your family's physical fitness. Is your daily dietary intake well balanced, and does it consist of plenty of nutrient-rich whole foods? Do you all get the recommended thirty to sixty minutes of daily exercise? Are you spending enough time together to support these important health goals?

The World Health Organization estimates that between 60 to 85 percent of the world's population leads a sedentary lifestyle, and the resulting lack of fitness may be among the ten leading global causes of death and disability. So if you aren't an active bunch, you aren't alone. The good news is that you have the chance to do something about it now.

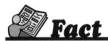 **Fact**

According to the U.S. Department of Health and Human Services, seven in ten American adults don't exercise regularly. Sedentary lifestyles are estimated to contribute to 300,000 preventable deaths annually from diseases such as heart disease, diabetes, and stroke.

For parents who were already eating nutritiously and exercising regularly, a fitness program would be nothing out of the ordinary— but perhaps it's a new concept to involve your children fully in your efforts. Maybe you work out at the gym daily, but you don't encourage physical activity during family time. Or maybe you eat healthful meals away from home while stocking your shelves with the deep fried, sugar-coated, trans-fatty snacks your kids always ask for. If so, it will be necessary to realign your personal fitness goals to take your child's needs into account as well.

Fostering Family Unity

Americans are busier than ever, but as a nation we are getting less exercise than ever before. That particular paradox is frequently what creates a weight issue in the first place. Between a parent's work and social obligations for parents, and the child's school commitments and extracurricular activities, it can be hard to find time to come together as a family. Sit down today and commit to at least one weekend day that you can designate as family time. If you work weekends or have other critical weekend commitments that just can't be moved, then choose at least two weeknights, weekday afternoons, or other time periods when your schedules align, and block them off for family use. More is of course encouraged, but for now make that minimum commitment.

Obviously when and how long you can spend time together will be variable, and your schedules may require readjustment as short-term events and commitments pop up. The important thing is to make an ongoing commitment to spending a specific amount of time together each week and sticking to it. It is insignificant if your family's together time falls on a Tuesday one week and a Thursday the next, as long as you make sure to find the time.

 Essential

> Households with two working parents, and those who work second or third shifts or alternating schedules, can leave little daylight time for family fitness. If your child spends many waking hours with a caregiver, it's imperative for that individual to get involved in exercise and nutrition routines.

If a look at your calendar makes you think that twice a month is a more realistic goal, you need what's commonly called a reality check. Really examine your own commitments, do the same for your child's, and then think about where adjustments can be made. Overextending yourself isn't good for you or your children. It may not be realistic to eliminate activities related to your job or workplace, but you may be able to scale back your social or community obligations. Or perhaps cutting back on time spent working is a feasible goal. Prioritize until you've carved out time for your weekly family togetherness commitment.

Lifestyle Makeover

Feeling overwhelmed by the prospect of overhauling your family's daily routine? Don't be. Remember that you don't have to change everything at once, and you may be surprised by how many positive routines your family already has in place. Start by assessing your habits—both good and bad—by keeping a family fitness log for a week. Write down all meals and snacks (including what, how much, and where) and physical activities. Everyone in the family should be part of the assessment. If some members are less than forthcoming with the information, do your best to estimate. Try not to interrogate; you'll only put family members on the defensive and probably won't get an accurate answer anyway.

Another approach is to give each member of the family a notebook to tally his or her own meals and activities. With this method, everyone is on the honor system. You should stress that this is a nonjudgmental exercise designed not to pick out individual faults, but to assess where you might improve your family routines.

Once you have a week's worth of family information logged, schedule a family meeting to sit down together and analyze your data. Look for trends, like meals being consistently skipped and family members eating in shifts rather than together.

Some additional questions to ask include the following:

- How many snacks and meals were eaten on the go or while performing other activities?
- Is your daily food intake roughly equivalent to the USDA recommended daily allowance for each food group? (See Chapter 6 for more information.)
- Does your daily diet contain plenty of fresh, whole foods, or is it mostly processed and packaged goods?
- Do you cook appropriate amounts and serve reasonable portions? Are you eating just until you're full or until the plate is clean?
- How much water are you drinking? Are your other beverages of choice full of empty calories?

- What kinds of meals are the kids getting at school? Do they have access to vending machines or other sources of candy and snacks at school or at extracurricular activities?
- Are the kids getting at least sixty minutes of moderate physical activity each day, and are the adults getting at least thirty minutes?
- How often does the family engage in physical activity together?

Once you've analyzed where your family is in terms of nutrition and exercise, it's time to set some goals for where you'd like to go together.

Setting Goals

Goals should *not* be a magic number on the scale. Instead, you should focus on changes you can make right now to work towards a healthier family. It's fine to start with smaller goals, such as eating your five-a-day servings of fruits and vegetables, walking your kids to school instead of driving, or packing a nutritious lunch for your child instead of sending money for corndogs and tater tots.

You should also have long-term goals established that include the nationally recognized standards for exercise and nutrition. That includes an hour of daily exercise for kids (thirty minutes daily for adults) and daily food intake that follows the USDA guidelines. No one—and no one family—is perfect, and while some weeks you may meet those objectives, there will be plenty of times you won't. The important thing is that they're always there to aspire to. Chapter 6 has more information on USDA standards and other nutrition issues, and Chapter 10 addresses exercise for children.

Don't Forget to Make It Fun

You don't want your children to start referring to your evening walk together as "the nightly death march." If they aren't enjoying an activity you choose for the family, by all means, try something different until you find one that they do. Let your children take turns choosing family outings. Roller- or ice-skating, snowboarding, bicycling, kayaking, canoeing, football, tennis, Frisbee, golf, bowling—the list is endless. Reluctant to plan a trip to the skating rink or to rent a canoe, just because you've never done it before? All the more reason to try these things out! You may find a new activity your child can be passionate about, or you may discover that it isn't your cup of tea, but at least you've had fun together trying it.

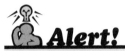

Alert!

Up to 40 percent of American families seldom eat together, despite abundant research pointing to the benefits of family meals. A 2003 Columbia University survey found that kids who ate with their families between five and seven times each week were 21 percent less likely to try tobacco and alcohol. A 2003 study published in the *Journal of Adolescent Health* found that adolescents who eat meals with their families four or five times weekly were significantly more likely to eat more vegetables, fruits, and dairy products.

Mixing It Up

Remember that you don't have to make a big financial investment in sporting goods or equipment to mix things up. Rentals are relatively cheap, and when even those may be a strain on the budget, you can find other ways to add entertainment value to less glamorous activities like family walks. Try some new locales, such as a local forest preserve or beach, and make your trek a nature hike. Add a list of items each child has to find on your journey, and you have a scavenger hunt. If your older children enjoy personal challenges, buy them an odometer for their bikes or a pedometer for their waistbands, and let them try to reach new distance goals with these activities. Whatever you choose to do, make it interesting and fun for your child. Don't hesitate to change gears if your current fitness plans are greeted with groans and rolling eyeballs.

One Size Does Not Fit All

Family fitness shouldn't be about keeping up with the Joneses, or even about keeping up with mom or dad. You and your children each have unique interests and abilities that you should encourage and nurture. Sometimes this will involve tailoring your fitness routines to accommodate these differences.

It's possible that dad's bad knee makes ice-skating a bad choice, while mom's fear of heights has her wary of a day on the ski slopes. Split up some family activities to accommodate different physical needs and interests. Mom may take one child skating while the other skis with dad. Later that day or even at the next family outing, the kids can switch places.

Adapting to family members' special needs is also important in the dietary arena. When your child has food allergies and your spouse is on a cholesterol- or sodium-restricted diet, you have those added needs to consider when balancing your family food plan. The good news is that if you've already been paying careful attention to what your family is eating, you probably won't have as difficult an adjustment to planning healthy meals the whole family will enjoy.

Everyone's a Winner

Children who are not competitive or athletically inclined will start to dread family activities if they revolve around contests in which one person strives to be the best or beat the others. While the ages of your children will influence what activities you share in as a family, you should also remain aware that kids of similar ages may have very different levels of expertise at certain things. If this is an issue for your family, and your child seems to feel intimidated by a sibling's athleticism, be sure to focus family time on noncompetitive activities that can be enjoyed at a variety of fitness levels. Hiking, swimming, and cycling may be good fits for your family.

Be Flexible

Although its important to commit to regular family fitness time each week, also recognize that a particularly difficult homework assignment, an unplanned meeting at the office, a school play, or any other number of other happenings may occasionally get in the way of your family plans. Be willing to work with the schedule, and adjust it as necessary. You should make it clear, however, that all family members who can speak and plan their own social activities without parental involvement are responsible for letting you know about upcoming events so you can plan ahead. You can't rely exclusively on the memory of your younger children, but you can ask that they take responsibility to the best of their ability.

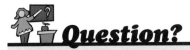 **Question?**

My kids have a knack for telling me about a scout meeting or a big game the morning of the event. How can I plan family time when things are so last-minute?
Keeping track of your younger child's calendar should be easy. Unless you pester them for details, however, older kids and teens don't always clue Mom or Dad in to important events until the last minute. At the start of each school week, ask your child if there are any important assignments or school-related events planned for the week, and note them on the family calendar. Encourage your kids to write in events on the calendar, too.

You should also remain flexible about what you're going to do and have options in mind should weather or other uncontrollable factors throw a wrench into your plans. When rain puts the kibosh on your biking adventure, a visit to the indoor community pool may be a backup plan.

Finally, flexibility is a must when trying to plan meals for picky eaters. Don't force-feed your child broccoli if she hates it, no matter how good it is for her. She can have carrots and green beans every night if those are the vegetables she knows and loves. That doesn't mean the rest of the family has to forsake the broccoli. You can also think about preparing broccoli in different ways for other family members—your picky eater may decide it looks pretty good after all in a different dish or form.

Providing a wide variety of tasty, nutritious foods is the best way to please a family that may have very different tastes. To keep yourself or your spouse from having to spend hours on end in the kitchen, give children their food choices before you prepare the meal. This way, you can ensure that they're going to eat at least something that's on the menu, and food won't go to waste.

When One Child Is Heavy

Heavy children with thin siblings may feel greater anxiety about their weight problem, particularly if a brother or sister engages in any teasing about size. Even the best kids can say hurtful things in a moment of heated sibling conflict. Do let your children know that name-calling and teasing will not be tolerated, and when it does occur, initiate any consequences immediately.

Sibling dynamics can also be complicated by feelings of jealousy and resentment. One child may feel jealous of all the extra attention he believes his sibling is getting as the family focuses on the weight-loss issue. On the other hand, your overweight child may be envious of his sibling because he doesn't have to "try" to lose weight. Again, focusing on healthy eating and activities as a family lifestyle change that will benefit all can help diffuse some of those feelings.

Challenges and Changes

No matter what their weight, all of your children can be challenged by your new lifestyle in some way. Perhaps your thin but inactive daughter will pick up a new sport or athletic skill that inspires her. Or maybe your son who enjoys cooking will come up with creative ways to serve up new healthful dishes.

Facing new challenges as a family will strengthen the bonds between child and parent and between siblings. Engage them in activities that set up a cooperative sibling spirit rather than a competitive one. A big brother or sister may be able to teach a younger sibling a skateboard trick or some new basketball shots. In addition to the health rewards your children will reap from this lifestyle shift, exposing him to new activities and new foods may spark his adventurous spirit and make him more willing to try new things in all areas of his life.

Avoiding Resentments

If sodas and sugar-laden snacks were once regular staples in your household, their sudden absence may be protested quite vocally. Your children who aren't struggling with a weight problem may find it easy to place blame for this edible embargo on their heavier sibling. Try to keep the blame card out of play up front by making it clear to your children that the changes you're instituting in your household are for the health of the entire family.

 Essential

If your kids are less than enthusiastic about their new way of eating, try piquing their interest with a culinary challenge to see who can create the healthiest and tastiest meal. Pair up younger children with an older sibling or parent, and let them take charge of everything from the grocery shopping to the presentation.

You may want to talk about how certain former snack favorites are poor choices for anyone—slim or heavy, young or old—due to their high content of trans fats or their nutrient deficits. Ensure you always have plenty of healthy snack choices on hand for all of your children to indulge in, such as fresh fruits, whole-wheat crackers, yogurt, and other favorites.

Be prepared for the inevitable questions about why they could eat this and that before and can't eat it now. Answer truthfully. Let your children know that you aren't perfect and that you're learning more about healthy foods just as they are. Explain that some of your former favorites are also on the unhealthy list, and while you may miss them at first, the health and strength you'll gain in the long run will more than offset those feelings.

Encouraging Empathy

Every parent wants their children to be considerate of the feelings and needs of others. Charity doesn't always begin at home, however, and kids will occasionally say things to their sisters or brothers that they'd never dream of saying to friends or even complete strangers. When they say hurtful things or complain about their siblings, remind them that you expect them to follow the Golden Rule—"Do onto others as you would have them do onto you." Ask how they would feel if they were on the receiving end of the same treatment they just dished out. Remember that your overweight child may not be blameless in the sibling wars either, so make sure you use an even hand in dispersing discipline and encouraging empathy.

When you see your children respecting the feelings of their siblings through words and actions, reinforce that behavior with praise and encouragement. Don't forget to practice what you preach—think about why a child who is usually kind is picking on his overweight sister. Are you focusing on her problems to the exclusion of his needs? Is he feeling uncertain about his role or importance in the family? Be an empathetic parent, and put yourself in each of your children's shoes.

Avoiding the Food Police Role

Autonomous control of when, how much, and what we choose to eat is something that is closely identified with our sense of independence from birth. An infant that wants to eat will make his needs known, loudly, and when fed he will eat until he is full. When solid foods start to be fed, a baby that doesn't like mashed turnips or chicken sticks will make his displeasure known instantly by ejecting them back at whoever sent them his way. Self-regulation of food intake is important for a child's sense of self-esteem, his independence, and for learning lifelong habits of healthy eating.

Remember, you are not the food police. Your job is to facilitate a healthy level of self-regulation, not to control every bite that goes into your child's mouth. Be a gatekeeper, providing healthy foods and educating your child on nutrition and fitness so he can make good decisions outside of the home. You can't be with your child around the clock, every day of the week, and even if you are now, you won't be forever. He needs input and control over his own fitness plan, so try your best to take a step back and let him steer the ship.

If you see him eating something he shouldn't, don't interrogate or nag. Think about how the scene has unfolded and what you can do to prevent it from happening again. First of all, is it a food item that you have around the house but shouldn't? Have you provided other appropriate and tasty options that he could have chosen from instead? When your child seems to be eating inappropriately because he had a particularly bad day at school or is feeling down, encourage him to talk about the problem instead of finding comfort in food. Let him know you are there for support so the next time he can run to you instead of the refrigerator.

Educating the Extended Family

Your child has been working hard at her fitness program, eating well and feeling good about her progress. Then she spends the weekend at her grandparents' house, where cooking comfort food—and eating the creations—is an Olympic event. After chocolate chip pancakes, home fries and hoagies, and a film festival with soda by the gallon and a barrel full of butter-drenched popcorn, she comes home either depressed about the setback or defiant that her grandparents "love her enough" to give her the foods she craves but you don't.

Staying on Track Away from Home

Hopefully, any extended family members or close friends who may play host to your child will be supportive of your family fitness goals and will provide an atmosphere where your child can continue her new lifestyle just as if she were at home. But even if they don't understand or believe in what you're doing, there are still some ways to ensure that your child can continue her progress when she's on someone else's turf. Here are a few suggestions:

- **Be proactive.** Let them know ahead of time that your child is on a fitness program, and outline her dietary and activity needs very clearly in writing.
- **Have carry-in.** Send along foods and beverages that are on your child's menu plan. If the host likes to cook, offer some healthful recipes as well.
- **Keep it low-key.** You don't want to make your child's diet the center of attention and make her feel self-conscious. Speak with the adults in private and let them know she's trying to be healthier.
- **Take a hard line on health.** Grandparents and other relatives will be less likely to dismiss your dietary requests as too strict if you emphasize that your child's doctor thinks they are necessary.
- **Suggest substitutions.** Let them know what healthy options are acceptable so they have suitable foods to offer your child.
- **Encourage activity.** If your kids go into coach-potato mode when they visit the grandparents, ask that television time be limited.

In some cases, your child's grandparents or other older relatives or friends may have physical limitations that keep them from going on long walks or participating in other activities. Usually all it takes is a little creative thinking to get past this obstacle. You can suggest that your child do some yard work, gardening, or other active chores for their host. Walking the dog or washing the car are also good ways to get out and about. If there are other children in the neighborhood close to your child's age, she may be able to enjoy some outdoor playtime with them.

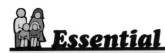
Essential

When your child stays with relatives or friends to celebrate a holiday or special occasion, you don't want him to overdo it on rich foods and desserts. At the same time, you don't want him facing a plate of carrot sticks while everyone around him has cake and ice cream. Let his hosts know that he can partake in some party fare as long as it's in moderation. See Chapter 14 for more information on handling special occasions.

Love and support from extended family and friends will go a long way in helping your child achieve her fitness goals, so take the time to educate those around her appropriately.

CHAPTER 5

Weight Loss 101

In theory, weight loss is simple. All you have to do is to make sure your child burns more calories than he consumes. But as you already know, perhaps from personal experience, it's not that easy. Metabolism, hormonal changes, social and psychological factors, and personal and family motivation all play a role, making weight loss anything but an uncomplicated process. As your child develops physically and matures emotionally, his fitness needs will change too. Parental guidance remains important to keeping both weight and well-being on track.

The Biology of Weight Loss

The only way for your child to get rid of excess weight is to use more calories than he eats. If his calorie intake is above what his body requires for daily activity and physical growth, and he doesn't use that energy for exercise or other activity, those bonus calories have to go somewhere. His body will take that extra fuel and store it as fat. Conversely, if he cuts his daily calories (or keeps them steady) and increases activity levels, his body will turn to those fat stores for energy.

The rate of your child's metabolism will also impact how quickly, or slowly, he loses weight. In addition, hormonal changes (such as those that hit at puberty) also play a role. How many calories your child should take in is based on his age and gender. **Table 5-1** outlines the suggested daily caloric requirements for girls and boys by age as rec-ommended by the U.S. Department of Agriculture (USDA).

As of the writing of this book, the USDA's Center for Nutrition Policy and Promotion was in the process of developing a revised ver-sion of the USDA food pyramid. The information provided here on daily calorie requirements for children is based on the daily food intake patterns that the food pyramid uses as its foundation. Because the new food pyramid will not be finalized until 2005 (after this book has gone to press), you'll find both the current and the proposed caloric standards below (Tables 5-1 and 5-2, respectively). The pro-posed energy requirements for daily food intake in the new food pyramid are based on the Institute of Medicine's *Dietary Reference Intakes Report* (2002).

Please note that any new information regarding the food pyra-mid that is included here is based on the proposed preliminary draft data from the USDA as of early May 2004 and does not reflect any changes made after the point. As such, the information provided here may turn out to be different from the final published release. Always consult with your child's doctor and/or her registered dietitian for the most current official dietary standards and how they apply to your child's particular health situation.

Table 5-1: Daily Energy (Calorie) Requirements (as of May 2004)		
Age Range	**Females**	**Males**
1–3	1300	1300
4–6	1800	1800
7–10	2000	2000
11–14	2200	2500
15–18	2200	3000

Table 5-2: Daily Energy Requirements (projected, 2005)			
Age range	Activity level	Females	Males
2–3	Sedentary	1000	1000
	Low active	1000–1200	1000–1400
	Active	1000–1400	1000–1400
4–8	Sedentary	1200	1400
	Low active	1400–1600	1400–1600
	Active	1400–1800	1600–2000
9–13	Sedentary	1600	1800
	Low active	1600–2000	1800–2200
	Active	1800–2200	2000–2600
14–18	Sedentary	1800	2200
	Low active	2000	1400–2800
	Active	2400	2800–3200

Sedentary indicates no regular exercise outside of the daily physical activities of living. Low active means regular exercise equivalent to walking 1.5 to 3 miles daily at a rate of approximately 3 to 4 miles per hour. Active is regular exercise equivalent to walking more than 3 miles daily at 3 to 4 miles per hour.

The 3500-Calorie Equation

Calories in food are actually measured in kilocalories—the amount of energy required to raise the temperature of one kilogram of water by exactly 1°C. Fats are high in calories, while proteins and carbohydrates are lower. (One gram of fat has nine calories, and proteins and carbohydrates have four calories per gram each.)

To lose one pound of body weight, your child needs to burn 3,500 calories more than he consumes. That goal is best reached through a combination of dietary and exercise adjustments. A fitness diary that tracks diet and activity can help you determine if he's eating more calories than required for his age. Just adding a brisk one-hour family walk to your child's routine can burn an extra 440 calories daily and could potentially add up to a total weight loss of six pounds per year without any adjustments in calorie intake.

Remember that the best types of calories to cut back on are those that are low in nutrients. Chips, soda, candy, anything deep-fried—it isn't hard to find suitable targets for elimination in the modern American diet.

Metabolism

Metabolism refers to the chemical and cellular changes within the body that are associated with both generating and utilizing energy. When a substance introduced into the body (such as food or medicine) is metabolized, it is broken apart and processed for use in physical functions and growth. The human body needs a minimal number of calories just to perform the basic functions of living (for instance, breathing, pumping blood, maintaining the central nervous system functioning, and staying warm) throughout the day. That number is called the basal metabolic rate, or BMR (also known as resting energy expenditure, or REE). Up to 70 percent of the energy your child requires daily is for these basic needs.

Severely overweight children actually have a higher BMR than normal-weight children because their body mass is larger, and as a result they require more energy to fuel organ systems and basic bodily functions. **Table 5-3** provides the simple formulas for calculating BMR.

Table 5-3: Basal Metabolic Rate (BMR)		
Age range	**Female**	**Male**
0–3	(61.0 × weight) – 51	(60.9 × weight) – 54
3–10	(22.5 × weight) + 499	(22.7 × weight) + 495
10–18	(12.2 × weight) + 746	(17.5 × weight) + 651

Weight is in kilograms; one kilogram is equivalent to 2.2 pounds.

Source: The Commission on Life Sciences of the National Academy of Sciences, Recommended Daily Allowances *(1989).*

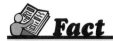 **Fact**

> Hormonal changes can impact basal metabolism. For example, the BMR starts to climb each month before women (and girls) get their menstrual period and then declines shortly thereafter. At puberty, as boys start to develop more muscle and girls more fat tissue, the average male BMR is approximately 10 percent higher than the female BMR.

The BMR can help you determine the bare minimum number of calories required to sustain a sleeping or completely still child. But since no child sits still for very long, you also need to know your child's active metabolic rate (or AMR). This is the caloric requirement for a day's worth of all physical activity (including everything from getting dressed to running a marathon). Very active children may burn up to twice as many calories as their BMR.

Exercise naturally boosts your child's metabolism by calling on stored calories for fuel. The metabolic lift of physical exercise also continues up to an hour after the activity has ended. The other metabolic plus of exercise is that it builds muscle tissue. Muscle tissue needs more "fuel" to function—even when your child is at rest. Fat, on the other hand, isn't as active. By adding lean muscle mass to his body, your child will make use of calories much more readily.

Any calorie reduction in your child's diet should be incremental and moderate. When you dramatically cut calories, the body's natural reaction is to slow metabolism to conserve energy. It goes into a pseudo-starvation mode and stockpiles those calories in the form of fat for later use. In addition, your child's developing body may lose access to important nutrients. While some temporary weight loss may be achieved, the sense of deprivation your child experiences will not build the kind of life-long weight maintenance skills you want to encourage.

Metabolism is also impacted by weight gain. As body fat increases, your child's metabolism will slow to achieve what is called a "set point" or new (and higher) level of calorie/energy balance. The best way to keep your child's metabolism humming along efficiently is to encourage small and frequent meals, instead of one or two daily feasts. This way, the body will burn caloric energy as it is taken in throughout the day rather than getting it all at once and having to store the excess fuel in fat. Your child's metabolic rate will actually increase temporarily after eating as her body digests the food. Approximately 5 to 10 percent of the calories in the meal itself are burned during digestion/metabolism.

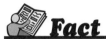 **Fact**

A child's metabolism is much faster than an adult's. Metabolism naturally slows down with age, although regular exercise can help speed things up again. Instilling healthy fitness habits in your child will serve him well throughout adulthood.

There are some endocrine disorders, such as Cushing's disease, that can impact metabolism and can cause excessive weight gain. Chapter 1 has more information on these rare but possible causes of overweight in children.

Hunger and Appetite

The appetite center of your brain is located in the hypothalamus. The lateral hypothalamus controls appetite signals, and the ventromedial hypothalamus controls satiety, or feelings of fullness. The hypothalamus is the master switch of the endocrine system, the hormone-secreting organs and glands that regulate such body functions as metabolism, growth, sexual development, and hunger.

Feelings of hunger and satiety are actually controlled by a self-regulating feedback loop that detects hormone levels in the bloodstream and secretes hormones in response. A complex series of biochemical processes mediate the relationship between hunger, metabolism, and weight in the brain. One enzyme (the AMP-activated protein kinase, or AMPK) helps "turn on" appetite. AMPK is activated when there isn't enough glucose energy present in the cells. The hormone leptin also operates on the hypothalamus, but with the opposite effect, suppressing appetite. However, studies indicate that people who are overweight or obese become resistant to leptin. PYY is another appetite-suppressant hormone that has been shown in human trials to reduce appetite by up to 30 percent. It appears not to cause resistance in the overweight as leptin does.

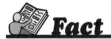 **Fact**

The hormone leptin, discovered in 1994, is secreted by fat tissue. It appears to achieve an appetite-suppressing effect by acting on neurons located in the hypothalamus. In animal studies, injections of the hormone transformed fat-storing cells into fat-burning cells. Adiponectin, another recently discovered fat-secreted hormone, was found to speed up metabolism and aid in weight loss in animals. Further research on these hormones may open doors for new weight-control treatment options.

Diet and Exercise: The Dynamic Duo

Cutting calories without adding activity is a recipe for eventual weight gain in children and adults alike. Your child's metabolism will recognize the game and slow down to conserve energy, resulting in a return of the weight and a more difficult time losing the pounds the next time around.

Fad diets promote the idea that weight loss is all about the food. Don't let your child get sucked into that line of thinking. Exercise is just as critical as food in efforts to reach a healthier weight. Encourage physical activity by making it fun—remember that most younger kids like to get out there and move.

As for the food, low-calorie, nutrient-dense fare is your child's best option. Try to limit "diet" foods that are heavy on preservatives and artificial sweeteners and light on protein, vitamins, and minerals. Healthy food choices are discussed in more detail in Chapter 6.

Getting Your Doctor's Help

Your child's pediatrician is an important ally in getting him on the track to good health. She can help you pinpoint the lifestyle factors (in rarer cases, the health or hormone problem) that are behind your child's weight issue and can also help you determine whether weight maintenance or weight loss is appropriate for your child. She can also screen for the existence of any weight-related health complications.

According to the U.S. Centers for Disease Control and Prevention (CDC), weight maintenance rather than weight loss is always the goal for children under two years of age. This approach allows them to "grow into" their weight and diminishes the possibility of caloric restriction depriving them of important nutrients needed for brain development and growth. The same strategy of weight maintenance goes for at-risk kids (those in danger of becoming overweight) and for those aged two to seven who are considered overweight but who aren't experiencing any weight-related complications (such as hypertension or high cholesterol).

Children who are candidates for gradual weight loss (of approximately one pound per month) include those with the following characteristics:

- Between the ages of two and seven, with a BMI in the 95th percentile or higher *and* the presence of weight-related complications
- Seven or older, with a BMI between the 85th and 94th percentile *and* the presence of weight-related complications
- Seven or older, with a BMI in the 95th percentile or above, *regardless of* the presence of complications

Potential health complications of childhood overweight issues are discussed in more detail in Chapter 1. In summary, however, these include hyperlipidemia (high cholesterol), hypertension (high blood pressure), glucose intolerance (prediabetes), insulin resistance, hepatic steatosis (fatty liver), cholecystitis (inflammation of the gallbladder), sleep apnea, and early puberty.

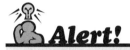

Alert!

A May 2004 study published in *The Journal of the American Medical Association* found that average blood pressure rates for children and teens have risen steadily since 1988, in part due to rising obesity rates. From 1988 to 1994, the average blood pressure of over 5500 American children surveyed was 104.6 over 58.4 (systolic over diastolic). In 1999–2000, it grew to 106 over 61.7.

Charting a Course

If your child's pediatrician believes weight loss is in order, the goal will be approximately one pound per month. That may not sound like a lot, but remember that your child is also growing taller and developing and will grow into at least some of the excess weight as time progresses. A conservative approach will ensure that she isn't losing weight too rapidly and is still getting the nutrients she needs for proper growth.

Goal Setting

Setting your child's sights on a magic number on the scale may backfire. While ideally you do want him to reach a healthy BMI for his age, it's more important that he look at this as a lifelong venture, not just a race to the finish line. Stay away from appearance- or popularity-related goals, and focus instead on gaining fitness skills. Here are some examples of healthy objectives:

- **Stay steady.** An initial goal for your child should be for him to not gain any further weight.
- **Feel better.** If your child's weight issues are causing medical complications such as orthopedic problems or sleep apnea, improving his health and well-being are important goals.
- **Energize!** Goals can be a simple as having enough energy to go on a challenging hiking or camping trip.
- **Go further and faster.** If your child gets winded when walking or is uncomfortable with long periods of activity because of the extra weight he's carrying around, ease of movement is a great incentive.
- **Personal best.** Some kids do find that reaching a new height in a challenging activity is just the push they need. The goal of walking the extra half-mile or swimming another two laps may be what they require to keep them focused.

Tracking Your Progress

A written log of your child's (and family's) progress towards their fitness goals can also help motivate, troubleshoot problem areas, and keep healthy living top of mind. To be effective, a food and fitness journal should be reasonably accurate, consistent, and detailed. Encourage complete honesty; let your child know that this is a tool, not a test, and no one will be punished for mistakes.

Food and Fitness Journals

Unless they're too young to write, kids should be responsible for keeping their own food diaries. A daily date book or planner will give your child a page for each day, which may serve as a good reminder for her. Any type of a notebook or journal will do, though. Let her pick it out if she'd like.

Journals are best kept in a chronological format and should include the following information:

- **Meals**—Everything your child eats at each meal of the day, along with where and when she eats the meal. Encourage your child to note when she has additional servings, and also to indicate if she was doing anything else (such as watching television) while eating.

- **Snacks (both big and small)**—All of your child's between-meal snack choices, and what time(s) of the day she snacks.
- **Drinks**—All beverages your child drinks, except for water.
- **Movement**—Exercise activities, both formal (like softball practice or gym class) and informal (walking to and from school, a bike ride to a friend's house).
- **Down time**—How much time your child spends watching television, playing video games, and participating in other sedentary activities.
- **Diary**—A space for personal reflections on what kind of a day your child had. These notes can help you determine when eating behaviors are tied to emotional or social cues.

Kids want and need their privacy, so if your child has qualms about sharing his journal with you, talk about it. You may be able to solve the problem by having him maintain the diary section of his journal in a separate place and giving him the option of sharing it with you only if he feels comfortable doing so. Ask only that he faithfully spend a few minutes doing it at the end of each day. Even if you never get the opportunity to see the diary portion, it will allow your child to start to consciously link his feelings and thoughts with his fitness behaviors.

Because you're all in this together, it's a really good idea to keep an ongoing family journal as well. As you work on instilling healthier behaviors, you should keep a journal that chronicles family meals and activities and your own observations on daily obstacles and victories. Try to include this information:

- **Meals**—List everything you put on the table for family meals, including condiments and drinks. If serving something new, note how it was received and how you might be able to improve upon the meal next time around. You can also include snacks if you'd like.

- **Family activities**—Make sure you include everything from yard work and chores to family walks and bike rides.
- **Grocery lists**—Keeping your grocery list in your fitness journal will keep healthy choices top of mind. It also allows you to keep running lists as you evaluate what new healthy foods were popular, and not so popular, with your family.
- **Achievements**—Did your child actually request fruit for a snack when she bounced in the door after school? Were the kids outside playing all day without so much as a mention of the television? Record the victories (big and small) that your family accomplishes.
- **Daily wrapup**—Similar to your child's diary section of her personal journal, the wrapup will allow you to jot a few notes about the day's events and the family's emotional temperature. If your child is keeping her diary private, then having your own record of things is even more helpful.

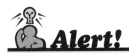

Alert!

Never go to the grocery store without a list. And once you're there, stick to the list! Impulse buys have been the downfall of many a fitness plan. Steer clear of the bakery, and don't go down aisles unless you need things there (to avoid unnecessary temptations). Finally, if it's at all possible, don't bring the kids. The relentless pleas for sugar-crusted breakfast cereals and other unhealthy favorites may wear down your resolve.

Keeping a food and fitness journal may seem arduous at first, but if you set aside ten to fifteen minutes at the end of each day to complete the task, it will soon be routine. Once you and your child are in the groove and keeping regular records, you should designate one hour a week for going over the results and looking for weaknesses and strengths. Appendix A has sample journal formats you can use.

Identifying Patterns and Problem Areas

Make the effort of analyzing your fitness journals a collaborative one. Encourage complete honesty, and really listen to your child—even if you don't always like what she has to say. If she tells you she hated the tofu surprise you served for dinner, for instance, you should not defend its nutritional value. Instead, talk about what other alternatives she might like you to try.

Quite a bit can be learned from where and when your child eats his meals. You may notice he eats twice as many after-school snacks on rainy days when he sits in front of the television than on days when he enjoys his snack outdoors. Skipping breakfast probably makes him ravenous for the wrong kinds of food at lunch. The very act of writing down his mealtime habits will make him more aware of the issues that influence his fitness. Talk about trends that you and your child notice as you do your weekly review.

Finally, always try to find something positive to say about the week, even when it's been a rough one for your child. Perhaps she passed up a fat-filled favorite at the school cafeteria, or maybe she walked home from school instead of taking the bus. Just the fact that she continued to write in her journal each day is reason enough to let her know you're proud of her commitment to her health.

Gold Stars: Kids and Motivation

Getting fit can be a long road with plenty of speed bumps along the way. Of course, telling your child that he's doing great is always important, and your encouragement will mean a lot to him—especially during the difficult times. But depending on his age and personality, reinforcing his achievements in other ways may also be necessary. Since kids aren't typically known for their vast reserves of patience, some rewards along the way may help maintain their enthusiasm and motivation.

Reward Systems: What Works and What Doesn't

Money can't buy you love, and it can't buy a healthy kid, either. So promises of a new bike, a trip to Disney World, or a new television for the bedroom aren't wise. First of all, if your child fails to meet the goal, he'll be devastated because the stakes were so high. Second, if he does meet the goal, you'll need to top the reward the next time around—because chances are you'll have to keep it up for your child to stay motivated.

On the other hand, small tangible incentives can be a valuable motivator for kids, especially young ones. The trick is to space them out and make them special. Ensure your child understands that while she has earned it through her efforts, the greatest reward is the achievement itself. A kind of frequent flyer program for kids works well, in which your child earns points for tasks related to her fitness. Keeping her fitness diary up to date without reminders or nagging, walking to school every day for a week, helping to cook a healthy family dinner—all these could be potential point earners. Sit down and assign point values to those tasks you think worthy (or those your child is having difficulty with), and then decide how many points it will take for a reward to be earned. Once you have a system in place, be consistent with it. If your child learns she can pester you into bending the rules, you've undermined the value of the program.

A Prize with a Purpose

As for the rewards themselves, keep the purpose of the program in mind. It goes without saying that food is not a good reward choice, and the use of food as a reward could be one of the causes behind weight gain in the first place. Better is something that provides a push towards your child's fitness goals—a special trip or event that is both fun and active. A trip to the zoo or beach, an afternoon of horseback riding, or a Saturday at the water slides. It doesn't have to be expensive, either. A backyard camping adventure or a ride to the best park in town are fun options that cost little to nothing.

If you must make the reward a gift or gadget, try items that encourage activity, too. A ball, a new bell for the bicycle, a butterfly net, or a plastic bucket full of beachcombing toys are all possibilities. Older kids might enjoy music that they can listen to on a personal stereo while walking, or a pass to the skating rink or swimming pool. Having some of these items stashed away for those days when the incentive is needed or the goal reached is a good idea; it can be too easy to forget a promised item or deliver it so late that the power of the incentive has been diminished.

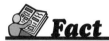 **Fact**

In the 1990s, University of Buffalo researchers began a series of studies on behavioral modification and weight loss in children. They found that overweight kids who were reinforced, or rewarded, for reducing preferred sedentary behaviors like watching television lost more weight than those who were restricted from those behaviors. The kids who were kept away from television and other sedentary pursuits also ended up liking those behaviors more than the kids who were rewarded for seeking alternative ways of entertaining themselves.

Motivation from Within

Adults often use negative motivations to work towards personal weight loss. You know the kind of thing—buying clothes two sizes too small, trying to fit into that pair of jeans from high school, or putting "fat pictures" on the refrigerator. These can backfire on adults, and they should never be tried on children. All these tactics send the message that "You're not good enough now." Your child needs positive motivation if he's going to achieve and maintain a healthy weight and fitness levels.

Of course, the best motivation for weight loss is a genuine drive from within to feel better and be healthy. But kids (and adults) are often motivated by appearance issues, emotional distress from peers, and the social stigma of being overweight in a society that places value on slim and trim. While you work with your child to improve his fitness level through dietary and activity changes, reinforce regularly that his size doesn't make him who he is. Once again, weight is a health issue, not an appearance issue.

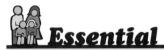 **Essential**

Set a good self-image example for your child. Do you refuse to get your picture taken ("I'll break the camera!"), have a hard time accepting a compliment ("Thanks, but I look awful today"), or repeatedly mention how inadequate you are ("I look fat in this")? Stop the negative talk, and try to say something positive to counter it each time you slip and criticize yourself. Your child will follow your example.

And what about the child who appears to be perfectly happy (if not healthy) at her current weight? First of all, be thankful you have a self-assured child who is confident in her appearance. That's often harder to achieve than weight loss itself. Make sure you don't undermine that confidence by sending the signal that she isn't okay "as is." Again, focus on the health issues, and make this a family move toward fitness that she is just one part of. If she sees that everyone is working towards more activity and eating healthier foods, she won't feel singled out or start to question her appearance. For more on making fitness relative, see Chapter 4.

When Slipups Happen

Everyone falls off the wagon once and a while. Put yourself in your child's shoes. When you've slipped up on a diet or an effort to kick a bad habit, did nagging or anger from the people you love help you or make the fall that much harder? And if yelling and screaming from a loved one did make you resolve to succeed once and for all, did your self-esteem or your sense of security in the relationship suffer at all?

Yelling, nagging, punishing, and using guilt simply don't work in any positive way to help your child when he stumbles. They may scare him into compliance temporarily, but in the long term these tactics do more harm than good. He may question his sense of value to you or shift his motivation for fitness to doing it for you instead of for himself.

If you see your child's empty ice cream bowl in the sink or find that she spent her lunch money on fast food again, take a minute to collect your thoughts, and rein in any frustration. Sit down and talk with her in a nonjudgmental way about what might have triggered the lapse. The reply "I don't know" is common and probably truthful, so ask specific questions. Were the alternatives available to her unappealing? Did she have a stressful day? If you can pinpoint a cause, you're more likely to prevent it, together, next time around.

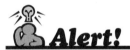

Alert!

A slipup can rapidly devolve into a binge if it isn't addressed appropriately. Your child may be upset or angry with herself, and those feelings are perfectly valid. A good way to get her back on track and provide a physical and emotional boost is to get out and move together—a brisk walk, a game of ball, or a bike ride. It's also a good opportunity to talk about possible triggers and address them.

The one situation that you are justified in being upset or even handing down a punishment with is if your child lies or uses deceptive tactics to try to cover up the dietary slipups. Sit down and have a talk with him, focusing on the fact that it's the deception you're upset and disappointed about and not the lapse in his meal plan.

Pushing Past Plateaus

When adults reach a point where weight loss levels off and they haven't reached their target goal, it's called hitting a plateau. For most kids it's a bit different. Unlike adults, children are continually growing taller and developing. So a stalled scale signals weight is being maintained. As kids grow up, they'll "fit" their weight better.

But some kids can hit their own kind of fitness plateau. One minute everything is going along fine, and they're maintaining or slowly losing extra weight; the next, they've gained a pound or two even though they're eating well and keeping active and a close examination of the fitness journal doesn't reveal any problems. Here are a few questions to ask:

- **Is it muscle?** If children have been lifting weights or doing any other sports that might tone or bulk their muscle mass, the weight could be coming from there. Muscle weighs more than fat.
- **Is it puberty?** Girls and boys will gain weight at puberty— boys in muscle mass and girls in fat tissue (unfair but true).
- **Is it a growth spurt?** Kids don't grow at a slow and steady rate. If they're weighing more, they could very well have picked up some height, too.

First of all, remind your child that it's how he feels that matters, not what the scale says. If this weight-loss plateau turns out to be the result of one of these transient causes, then the situation will soon resolve itself. If you can't pinpoint a problem and your child's weight continues to climb, however, it is time to make an appointment with your child's pediatrician to make sure there isn't a medical reason for the gain.

CHAPTER 6

Eating Right: Food Facts

H ow big is a serving? What's the right kind of fat, and how can you find out if a food has it? Does your child need a vitamin supplement? When faced with the task of healthy menu-planning, a good education in the essentials is a must. So is the help of a qualified dietitian, a few good books, and even some software if you're so inclined. No one said getting into the healthy eating routine was going to be easy, but once you have the basics down you'll be navigating the nutritional jungle in no time.

Who Makes the Rules, and What Are They?

So what's in the food your child is eating, and how do you know if it's healthy or not? If you've picked up a newspaper or flipped on the television recently, you've probably heard some new report on what food causes cancer or what nutrient prevents it. The result is often information overload, and without a basic education (or refresher course) in the nutrients, vitamins, and minerals your child needs, a trip to the grocery store or a session of menu-planning can leave your head spinning.

Although labeling laws have improved significantly in the past fifty years, all of the acronyms and mysterious-sounding nutrients (alpha-linolenic acid, anyone?) makes cutting through the jargon difficult. Here are a few acronyms you need to know:

- **RDA**—Recommended dietary allowance, or the average daily dietary intake level that meets the nutritional requirements of the majority (97 to 98 percent) of healthy people in a given demographic (such as female adolescents between fourteen and eighteen or children ages three to six).
- **DV**—Daily value. The DV is based on the RDA. It's used on the nutrition facts label to indicate what percentage of the recommended daily amount of a specific nutrient a serving of food provides. This term replaces the old "USRDA" (see below).
- **DRV**—Daily reference value. Dietary references for fat, saturated fat, cholesterol, carbohydrate, protein, fiber, sodium, and potassium based on a 2,000 calorie and 2,500 calorie diet.
- **RDI**—Reference daily intake. Average dietary reference values for vitamins, minerals, and protein (not age or gender specific). Formerly called "USRDA" (U.S. recommended daily allowances).
- **USRDA**—Obsolete term that signified the U.S. recommended daily allowances. Eliminated from food labels in 1994 so as not to be confused with the regular RDA (above). Has been replaced by DV.
- **DRI**—Dietary reference intake. Reference values established by the National Academies of Science that are used for planning and assessing nutrient intake for healthy people.
- **DRI 2002**—*Dietary Reference Intakes for Energy, Carbohydrate, Fiber, Fat, Fatty Acids, Cholesterol, Protein, and Amino Acids*, a report issued by the National Academies of Science (NAS).

Chapter 8 includes step-by-step descriptions for how to decipher a nutrition facts food label.

Setting the Guidelines: An Important Note

Nutrition and Your Health: Dietary Guidelines for Americans (known as *Dietary Guidelines for Americans*), a joint report of the U.S. Department of Health and Human Services (HHS) and the Department of Agriculture (USDA), is the basis for all federal food and nutrition policy. Based on scientific research, and updated every five years to incorporate the newest studies and findings, these guidelines are also used for nutritional guidance in the clinical practice of registered dietitians and health-care providers.

As of mid-2004, the HHS and the USDA were in the process of developing the sixth edition of their publication, along with a new graphic representation of the USDA food pyramid. One of the goals for the new edition is to incorporate the *Dietary Reference Intakes for Energy, Carbohydrate, Fiber, Fat, Fatty Acids, Cholesterol, Protein, and Amino Acids (DRI 2002)*, a report issued by the Food and Nutrition Board of the Institute of Medicine (part of the NAS) in 2002.

Therefore, information from *Dietary Guidelines for Americans* included in this chapter reflects the most current edition available as of the writing of this book (2000). Because the upcoming sixth edition will most likely incorporate the *DRI 2002* report recommendations, findings from that report are also included.

Carbohydrates and Fiber

Carbohydrates (or "carbs," for short), sometimes called sugars or starches, are the human body's main source of glucose. Once carbs are converted to glucose and enter the bloodstream, the pancreas secretes the hormone insulin, which enables the body's cells to use the glucose for energy. Glucose is also essential for central nervous system functioning.

Fiber is considered a carbohydrate, but unlike sugars and starches, it doesn't have an appreciable impact on blood sugar levels. When you're looking at the nutrition facts label on packaged food, you'll see that dietary fiber is included in the total carbohydrates listed, but is also broken out as a separate measurement so you can see how fiber-rich the food is.

Fiber is beneficial to both children and adults for a number of reasons. First of all, fiber doesn't break down significantly in the gastrointestinal tract. That makes it bulky and therefore filling. So a little bit of fiber goes a long way towards making you feel full. Second, fiber promotes both heart and gastrointestinal health. Insoluble fiber, found in whole grains like wheat bran and fibrous vegetables, keeps the colon clean, while soluble fiber—found in beans, berries, nuts, and seeds—soaks up the bile acids that convert to cholesterol.

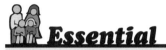 *Essential*

Sugar is a carbohydrate, and it is included in the "Total Carbohydrates" entry on the nutrition facts label. Sugar is also listed separately, along with fiber, underneath the carb total so you can see how much added sugar the product contains. The USDA recommends that sugar intake should be limited. The *DRI 2002* specifies that total daily sugar should be less than 25 percent of daily calories.

Recommendations for Total Carbohydrates

The USDA- and FDA-recommended daily value for carbohydrates is 60 percent of total calories. *DRI 2002* recommends that 40 to 65 percent of daily calories come in the form of carbohydrates. For children between age one and eighteen, the RDA for carbohydrates is 130 grams.

Some clinical studies have indicated that regularly consuming high glycemic index carbs can reduce good cholesterol, increase bad cholesterol, and raise long-term blood glucose levels. Yet it is also unhealthy to consume too few dietary carbohydrates each day, as the body needs carbohydrate-generated fuel to function properly. See Chapter 7 for more information on the glycemic index of carbohydrates and controlled-carb and low-carb diets.

Recommendations for Fiber

Look for whole-grain breads and cereals, such as bran, which are kid-friendly and versatile food choices with plenty of fiber. Other good sources of dietary fiber include fresh fruits (with the skin on), popcorn, brown rice, and root vegetables. Children and adults should have 20 to 35 grams per day.

The *DRI 2002* recommends that children between the ages of one and three maintain an average intake of 19 grams of fiber daily. For children four to eight, the recommendation is 25 grams daily. Boys aged nine to thirteen should be eating 31 grams of total fiber each day; from ages fourteen to eighteen, they should have 38 grams daily. Girls from age nine to eighteen should consume 26 grams of total dietary fiber daily.

Fats and Cholesterol

Saturated fat, dietary cholesterol, and trans fatty acids (or trans fats) all raise blood cholesterol levels and the risk of heart disease, which is why their use should be limited. Unsaturated fats raise "good" cholesterol (HDL) levels while lowering bad (LDL) cholesterol levels, making them heart protective. Unsaturated fats are either polyunsaturated or monounsaturated, depending on their chemical structure. **Table 6-1** has information on what fats are found in what foods. Remember that all fats are high in calories, so even unsaturated fats should be used in moderation.

Table 6-1: Sources of Dietary Fat and Cholesterol	
Saturated Fats	
Foods High in Saturated Fats	Better Choices
Whole milk and full-fat cheese and ice cream	Lower-fat or fat-free versions; frozen yogurt
Butter, lard, and tropical oils	Unsaturated cooking oils like olive and sunflower, liquid margarines or spreads free of trans fats
Fatty cuts of meat and poultry skin	Leaner beef cuts, poultry with skin removed

Table 6-1: Sources of Dietary Fat and Cholesterol (continued)

Dietary Cholesterol

Foods High in Cholesterol	Better Choices
Egg yolks	Egg whites only, or EggBeaters (Note: Egg yolks are fine in moderation, since they contain vitamins A, D, and E.)
Full-fat milk, cheese, and ice cream	Lower-fat or fat-free versions; frozen yogurt
Liver and other organ meats	Skinless poultry or lean cuts of beef

Trans Fatty Acids (Trans Fats)

Foods High in Trans Fats	Better Choices
Some baked goods and chips	Products without hydrogenated or partially hydrogenated fats listed on the label
Some margarines and shortenings*	Unsaturated oils or those margarines labeled as being free of trans fats
Some fried fast foods	Cook at home in unsaturated oils, or opt for grilled menu choices

Unsaturated Fats

Sources of Unsaturated Fat

Fatty coldwater fish (such as salmon, tuna, mackerel, sardines)**

Vegetable-based oils (such as sunflower, safflower, canola, soybean)

Nuts and nut oils (such as almonds, peanuts, hazelnuts, walnuts, pecans)

Flaxseed and flax oils

Avocados

*In general, the more liquid the margarine or spread, the fewer trans fats it contains.

**Fish are an excellent source of omega-3 fatty acids. However, they can also be high in methylmercury, which can be neurotoxic to the central nervous system of young children and fetuses. Therefore, the FDA and EPA recommend that fish consumption of young children and pregnant women be no more than twelve ounces weekly and should exclude swordfish, king mackerel, shark, and tilefish.

Omega-3 Fatty Acids

Both children and adults should have a regular dietary source of omega-3 fatty acids. These essential dietary components lower heart-disease risk and may play a role in the treatment of some mental disorders. The omega-3 fatty acids include alpha-linolenic acid (ALA), eicosapentaenoic acid (EPA), and docosahexaenoic acid (DHA). ALA is found in green leafy vegetables, flaxseed and flaxseed oil, canola oil, soybean oil, walnuts, and Brazil nuts. EPA and DHA are found in coldwater fish and in fish oil. DHA is also found in breast milk. It is essential to an infant's brain and eye development.

Recommendations

The *Dietary Guidelines for Americans* recommends that total daily fat intake be limited to 30 percent of calories or less, with no more than 10 percent of that being saturated fats. Cholesterol should be limited to 300 mg daily. The *DRI 2002* recommends a slightly broader range for total fat intake—between 30 to 40 percent of daily calories for children between one and three, and between 25 to 35 percent for those between four and eighteen. There is no specified limit for saturated fat and cholesterol.

Protein

Dietary protein helps build muscles, maintain organ function, and is essential for your child's growth and development. Protein is either complete (meaning that it provides all of the nine amino acids, or building blocks of protein, that the body cannot produce on its own), or incomplete (meaning that it lacks one or more of the essential amino acids). Meat, eggs, fish, and milk are considered sources of complete protein, while fruits, vegetables, and grains have incomplete proteins. Both complete and incomplete proteins are part of a well-balanced diet, and incomplete protein sources can be combined to meet the total essential amino acid requirements of the body.

Recommendations

The reference daily intake (RDI) for protein for infants up to one year is 14 grams, and for children aged one to four the RDI is 16 grams. For those aged four and older, and for adults, a daily value for protein is set at 10 percent of total calories. The *DRI 2002* suggests that young children have a daily protein intake of 5 to 20 percent of total calories, while older children consume protein levels equivalent to 10 to 30 percent of the day's calories.

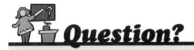 *Question?*

My son puts salt on everything. Does it hurt to spice things up a bit, or should I hide the shaker?
One teaspoon of table salt contains about 2300 mg of sodium. In addition, many processed foods, like chips and soups, are high in sodium. It isn't hard to exceed the recommended daily sodium intake of 2400 mg or less. Try offering salt alternatives, such as one of the many herb and spice blends available (check the label for hidden sodium), and encourage your son to sample before he seasons—he may be reaching for the shaker out of habit rather than for taste concerns.

The Food Pyramid

Most dietitians base their suggestions on the dietary requirements outlined in the USDA food pyramid and the food pyramid for young children, considered the foundation for good nutrition. The pyramid calls for the following daily servings (children aged two to six should eat the minimum number of servings):

- **Bread, cereal, rice, and pasta**—Six to eleven servings
- **Vegetables**—Three to five servings
- **Fruits**—Two to four servings
- **Milk, yogurt, and cheese**—Two to three servings

- **Meat, poultry, fish, dry beans, eggs, and nuts**—Two to three servings
- **Fats, oils, and sweets**—Use sparingly

In general, the lower range of servings is for people who are sedentary (or very young), while the higher range is designed to meet the caloric energy needs of more active individuals.

Legumes, or dried beans and peas, actually fit into two places in the food pyramid—the vegetables group and the meat, poultry, fish, dry beans, eggs, and nuts group. However, you should use the either/or method in figuring out their contribution. In most cases, they count towards your vegetable requirement; vegetarians and vegans, however, would count legumes in the meat category. The exception is if you eat multiple servings of legumes in a single day; once the vegetable requirement is fulfilled, you can count them towards the meat group, and vice versa.

Note that a serving on the food pyramid and a serving listed on a food label aren't necessarily equivalent (see the section titled "Dishing It Out," on page 88). **Table 6-2** gives USDA-mandated serving sizes from the *Dietary Guidelines for Americans*.

Table 6-2: USDA Food Pyramid Serving Sizes*	
Food Group	**Serving Size**
Bread, Cereal, Rice, and Pasta Group	1 slice of bread
	1 cup of ready-to-eat cereal
	½ cup of cooked cereal, rice, or pasta
Vegetable Group	1 cup of raw leafy vegetables
	½ cup of other vegetables, cooked or raw
	¾ cup of vegetable juice
Fruit Group	1 medium whole fruit (such as an apple or banana)

Table 6-2: USDA Food Pyramid Serving Sizes* (continued)

Fruit Group	½ cup of chopped, cooked, or canned fruit
	¾ cup of fruit juice
Milk, Yogurt, and Cheese Group**	1 cup of milk or yogurt
	1 cup of milk or yogurt
	1 ½ ounces of natural cheese
	2 ounces of processed cheese
	1 cup of soy-based beverage fortified with calcium
Meat, Poultry, Fish, Dry Beans, Eggs, and Nuts Group***	2 to 3 ounces of cooked lean meat, poultry, or fish
	1 to 1 ½ cups of cooked dry beans or tofu
	2 to 3 eggs
	5 to 7 ½ ounce soy burger
	4 to 6 tablespoons of peanut butter
	⅔ to 1 cup of nuts

*For children two to three years old, who require a lower overall energy intake, one serving is two-thirds of the standard serving sizes listed here. The exception is the dairy group, whose serving sizes are uniform regardless of age.

**Includes nondairy milk alternatives. Milk and dairy choices should be low-fat or fat-free, except for children age two and under.

***Includes meat substitutes.

Fluid Foundations

Adequate fluid intake will help cool off your child, promote healthy skin, keep all of her organ systems running smoothly, and prevent constipation. Many foods have a high water content (such as soup, watermelon, or grapes), and on average, food sources contribute to about one quarter of your child's daily fluid intake needs. The National Academies of Science recommend that children between the ages of one and three should be consuming at least 1.3 liters (about 44 ounces, or five and a half eight-ounce glasses) of water *from both beverages and foods* daily. Between ages four and eight, 1.7 liters (just over seven glasses, or 56 ounces) is recommended, and from age nine to thirteen, 2.4 liters (about ten glasses, or 80 ounces) for boys and 2.1 liters (just under nine glasses, or 72 ounces) for girls is the guideline. From ages fourteen to eighteen, boys need 3.3 liters daily (almost fourteen glasses, or 112 ounces) and girls require 2.3 liters (just under ten glasses, or 80 ounces).

Beware of beverages that are primarily sugar. Soda pop is an obvious offender, but many fruit juices also contain little fruit and abundant calories in the form of added sugars. The American Academy of Pediatrics recommends that juice intake be limited to four to six ounces for kids between one and six, and eight to twelve ounces for those seven and older.

Two of the healthiest drink choices are water (or noncaloric flavored waters) and low-fat or skim milk. Limit your child's consumption of sports drinks like Gatorade to activity times, during and after sports and exercise. While these drinks contain electrolytes that can prevent dehydration, they're also sugar-rich and shouldn't be a primary drink choice for inactive times.

Vitamins and Supplements

A varied diet is the best source of essential vitamins and minerals. Vitamins and minerals in food are better absorbed than the bottled variety, and they taste a whole lot better, too. If your child's diet is lacking in specific nutrients, either due to dietary patterns (such as vegetarianism or refusal to eat certain foods) or a health condition, your pediatrician may recommend supplements. Never give your child supplements without first consulting a doctor, as too much of some vitamins and minerals can be detrimental to a child's health.

Some important vitamins and minerals in your child's diet include the components listed in the following sections.

Iron

Iron is important to both young children and to girls who have reached puberty. Adolescent girls need 15 mg of iron daily, compared to 12 mg for adolescent boys. Younger children require 10 mg of iron each day. Keep in mind that the body only absorbs about 20 percent of dietary iron (less if it's plant-based, versus animal-based). Combining iron with foods high in vitamin C can boost absorption, while mixing it with foods containing tannins (found in tea) or calcium can decrease absorption.

Calcium

Adolescents in particular need sufficient calcium for their developing skeletal system and should have 1,300 mg daily between the ages of nine and eighteen (about three servings from the milk, cheese, and yogurt group). Children ages four to eight should get 800 mg daily (two servings), and kids age one to three should have 500 mg (which can be found in two eight-ounce glasses of milk). If your child is lactose-intolerant or has milk allergies, you may need to find an alternate dairy-free and calcium-rich food to introduce to the diet, such as collard greens or another dark green, leafy veggie.

Vitamin A

Vitamin A is important to immune-system function and to cell growth. Children ages one to three need 1000 IU (International Units) of vitamin A daily, and those between the ages of four and eight require 1333 IU. From ages nine to thirteen, 2000 IU is the RDA, and from ages fourteen to eighteen the RDA is set at 3000 IU. Cheese, eggs, liver, and carrots are all good sources of vitamin A.

Vitamin C

Vitamin C is an antioxidant that assists in wound healing and oral health. It may also have heart-protective benefits. Between the ages of one and three, children should get 15 mg of vitamin C daily, and from ages four to eight, 25 mg is the RDA. Kids aged nine to thirteen should have an RDA of 45 mg. Boys fourteen to eighteen require 75 mg of vitamin C daily, while girls in that age range need only 65 mg daily. Citrus fruits, strawberries, broccoli, green peppers, and tomatoes all contain vitamin C.

Vitamin D

The American Academy of Pediatrics recommends a vitamin-D supplement of 200 IU per day for those children and adolescents "who do not get regular sunlight exposure, do not ingest at least 500 mL per day of vitamin-D–fortified milk, or do not take a daily multivitamin supplement containing at least 200 IU of vitamin D."

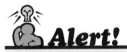

Alert!

Too much zinc can impair your child's immune system and cause decreases in HDL ("good") cholesterol, so talk to your pediatrician before considering a supplement with added zinc. From one to three years of age, zinc intake should not exceed 7 mg. The maximum intake for age four to eight is 12 mg, and children from age nine to thirteen should not have more than 23 mg of zinc daily. Adolescents fourteen to eighteen years of age should keep their daily zinc intake below 34 mg.

Zinc

Children seven months to three years of age should have 3 mg of zinc daily to ensure proper growth and immune system functioning. Between the ages of four and eight, children need 5 mg of daily zinc, and from ages nine to thirteen they need 8 mg. In adolescence, zinc requirements go up—boys need 11 mg, and girls need 9 mg through age eighteen. Most children can meet these requirements through diet—beef, oysters, fortified cereals, nuts, and beans are just a few of the foods rich in zinc.

Dishing It Out: Portion Control

One trigger for overeating in both children and adults is the tendency to pile too much on the plate. Over the past several decades, average portion sizes have climbed considerably for packaged foods, fast food, and on the restaurant menu. When faced with a beyond-heaping helping, many people do what comes naturally—they eat it, based on the "waste-not-want-not" theory and the "I'm getting my money's worth whether I'm hungry or not" principle.

Remember that your child can't handle adult-sized portions. Start small—a tablespoon or two of each dish—with the assurance that your child can have more if he wants it. Giving him a variety of healthful choices in small doses will also minimize food waste for those dishes he decides he doesn't care for.

Weighing in Portions

Keeping servings to appropriate sizes at home is an easy step towards fitness that you can implement today. It can also better equip you and your child to recognize overload when eating out. For packaged foods, the serving size is indicated right on the nutrition facts label. For meat, poultry, and fish, the average serving size is usually three ounces.

Since it isn't always practical to carry a kitchen scale around with you, following are a few typical serving sizes and points of reference for estimating portion sizes:

- Three ounces of fish, meat, or poultry is the size of a deck of cards or the palm of your hand.
- A cup of fruit or yogurt is the size of a baseball or a clenched fist.
- One teaspoon of butter or mayonnaise is the size of a thimble or a thumb tip (top knuckle to tip).
- One ounce of cheese is the size of an AA battery or your entire thumb.

The serving size on the nutrition facts label and the recommended serving size based on the USDA food pyramid are not always equivalent. Food pyramid serving sizes are based on portion sizes using standard household measures (such as a cup) and also on nutrient content in a serving. Nutrition facts serving sizes are based on a reference amount of food that is a typical portion based on data from national food consumption surveys. Sometimes servings are similar, and sometimes they aren't. Always check the label.

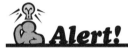

Alert!

A 20-ounce vending machine bottle of soda contains one serving, right? Wrong. Look at the nutrition facts closely, and you'll see that it actually contains two and a half 8-ounce servings. In this case, your child's calorie intake could have been more than twice what you might have assumed if you hadn't read the label carefully.

A 2003 study published in *The Journal of the American Medical Association* found that portion sizes of salty snacks, desserts, fruit and soft drinks, French fries, hamburgers, cheeseburgers, and Mexican food grew considerably from 1977 to 1998, both in the home and out at fast-food restaurants.

Preventing Portion Creep

From the grocery store to the kitchen table, there are plenty of ways to stop portions from growing out of control:

- **Downsize.** Buy small. If it's truly more economical to buy the large size, then have reusable containers or bags on hand and divvy the food up into sensible portions after you get it home.
- **Weigh in.** Invest in a kitchen scale and a set of wet and dry measuring tools.
- **Don't eat out of the bag.** Kids who snack directly from the bag

or box can't see how much they're really eating. Measure out a serving into a bowl instead.

- **Serve yourselves.** Let your kids dish out their own portions, and they'll most likely regulate the size more appropriately to their hunger than you will. If they tend to overdo it, tell them to start small and have seconds if needed.

Sharing meals and boxing half-helpings for home can help control your portions when eating out. For more on sensible and nutritious restaurant eating, see Chapter 9.

Quashing the Clean Plate Syndrome

Children know when they're full. Don't make cleaning the plate a requirement for leaving the dinner table. It's an arbitrary benchmark (especially if you dished up the meal to begin with). You'll only end up teaching your child to disregard their satiety signal, and he'll become accustomed to eating past his hunger. Using dessert as a reward for getting through a meal is also a bad idea for the same reason. In addition, it will set up your child to expect dessert every evening rather than as an occasional treat.

 Essential

How many calories your child needs daily is based on her age, gender, and activity level. Chapter 5 has detailed information on the caloric requirements of girls and boys by age and activity level. Use the nutrition facts label on packaged food to determine calorie count, and pick up a good calorie-counting book for fresh produce and other unlabeled items. If you like gadgets and can afford the price tag, there are food scales on the market that also calculate calories of a given helping.

Should you say no if your child says she's too full to finish her meal but then wants to have some of what the rest of the family is having for dessert? The best way to get around this dilemma is to always make dessert something nutritious rather than a sugar-splurge, like a fresh fruit salad or a fruit and yogurt parfait.

Menu Planning

Now that you know what foods your child should be eating on a daily basis, it's a good idea to try your hand at menu planning. Planning and shopping for a week's worth of meals will save you money and time and reduce the chance of impulse eating.

The best strategy is to see a registered dietitian (RD) first for guidance in setting your daily goals. If you haven't yet seen an RD or are waiting for your appointment, you can still do some general planning. Sit down and make a list of your family's favorites and those new dishes you'd like to try, and then consider how they fit within the food pyramid's daily serving guidelines. What sides can you add or substitutions can you make to bulk up the nutrient value? Remember that some foods may meet multiple requirements. For example, a soft taco fulfills servings in the grain, meat, vegetable, and dairy (if it includes cheese) groups. It's also a good idea to have your child's monthly hot-lunch schedule on hand if she eats at the cafeteria occasionally.

Once you have one day of a pyramid-friendly menu sketched out, see how it fits within the *Dietary Guidelines for Americans* and your child's calorie requirements. Remember that for each day, total fat should not exceed 30 percent of calories, and no more than 10 percent of that should be saturated fat. Total carbohydrates should not exceed 60 percent of calories, and total protein should not exceed 10 percent of calories. Don't forget to leave some leeway for healthy snacks, too. Then repeat the whole process for each day of the week.

Think about your family's schedule when deciding what meals to serve on what days. Extracurricular activities, appointments, and meetings at work may influence what you have and when you have it. It's also a good idea to have a few minimal muss-and-fuss options as backups should your schedule not go according to plan. Chapter

20 has tips for making the most of your money when menu-planning and food-shopping.

Consulting with a Dietitian

A family consultation with a registered dietitian (RD) is one of the best investments you can make in terms of your family's health. In addition to offering the latest nutrition education, an RD can help you with customized menu-planning strategies that fit your lifestyle and health goals and will appeal to a picky child or teen. For information on finding an RD, see Chapter 7.

Cookbooks, Software, and More

Even if you don't much like cooking, it will pay to stop by your local library or bookstore. Pick out several cookbooks with tasty-sounding recipes to add variety to your preparation of new dietary staples like fruits and veggies. The only requirements are that the recipes provide nutritional analysis, meet the needs of your family based on the *Dietary Guidelines for Americans,* use obtainable ingredients, and require a realistic amount of prep time for your lifestyle needs.

A printed guide that offers nutritional information on foods is also invaluable. Although the information is available for free online from the USDA, the published versions are much more manageable, portable, and readable. They frequently offer extra information on nutrients and cooking that makes them worth the extra dollars. Additionally, a growing number of chain restaurants are offering nutritional information on menu items either at their restaurants, online at company Web sites, or by request from corporate headquarters.

If there's a chef in your family, you may want to invest in a software program that offers nutritional analysis of a dish or an entire menu based on the recipes you use, such as AccuChef (Sivart), MasterCook (ValuSoft), The Living Cookbook (Radium Technologies), and Cook'n Software (DVO Enterprises). Many software packages have advanced features like scaling recipe yield for big crowds or small meals, generating an automatic shopping list, and long-term menu planning.

CHAPTER 7

Popular Diets: Separating Fact, Fad, and Fiction

W ith America's growing weight problems have come a slew of weight-loss plans and fad diets. From low-fat to low-carb and liquid to food combining, there's a diet out there that covers just about every gimmick and angle. While many may be good for some short-term weight loss, most popular diets lack one critical element for long-term success—balance. The best way to ensure that your child has the tools to develop healthy eating strategies to last a lifetime is to get professional nutritional counseling from a registered dietitian.

The "D" Word

You've pitched all the Ding-Dongs, Doritos, and Double-Stuffed Oreos and have loaded up the crisper to the brim with fresh fruits and veggies. Your bread is whole wheat, the freezer is full of fresh fish and lean meats, and there's not a marshmallow shape to be found in your new selection of breakfast cereal. "Let the diet begin!" you proudly proclaim. Time out. Your child and your family are *not* dieting. Don't even let that word—or the emotional and cultural baggage that travels with it—pass your lips.

Why "Diet" Is a Four-Letter Word
Once upon a time, "diet" was an uncomplicated concept with a simple definition—the typical types of food and drink a person regularly consumed. Occasionally,

we still use it in that context, but that's usually only when we're referring to nutritional requirements for a medical condition (such as a low-sodium diet for hypertension) or when talking about vegetarianism. Over the past century and a half, however, the American concept of "diet" has changed dramatically, implying food restrictions, deprivation, and limitations. In today's sense of the term, being "on a diet" means you are on a temporary quest for weight loss, not a long-range strategy for fitness through healthy food choices. That's exactly the type of thinking you want to discourage in your child or in your family.

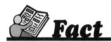 **Fact**

The first diet book, entitled *A Letter on Corpulence Addressed to the Public*, was published in the England by William Banting in 1863. Banting lost fifty pounds by eliminating sugar and starch from his diet and eating plenty of green vegetables, soft-boiled eggs, meat, poultry, and fish on the advice of his physician, William Harvey. Banting's book, which was essentially the first low-carb diet plan, was very popular in its time and went through several printings.

So refrain from using the "D" word when discussing your nutritional goals, and talk in terms of healthy foods and meal planning for fitness only.

Balance

Dieting seems to be one of America's favorite pastimes. From ultra low-fat to ultra low-carb and everywhere in between, the fad food plan of the moment frequently hinges on first demonizing and then dramatically reducing one major dietary component. But the human body, and especially the body of a growing child, needs abundant and varied sources of protein, carbohydrates, and healthy fats to thrive. That's why attempting to eliminate any one nutrient or category of nutrients from your child's food choices is never a good idea. Maintaining balance, and focusing on phasing out refined and highly processed junk foods in favor of whole fruits, veggies, and grains, is a winning strategy that will pay off longer than all of the bestselling diets of the moment combined.

Still, tales of rapid weight loss and dramatic downsizing may have you wondering about some of the popular plans behind the stories, and whether there's anything to them. There's a reason that the fine print with each testimonial invariably states "results are not typical." Yet beyond all the hype, there may be a thing or two to learn from the schools of thought behind today's most popular diet plans.

The Skinny on Low-Carb Diets

Unless you've been living under a rock for the past few years, you've heard a thing or two about low-carb diets like Atkins. Founded on the principle that it's excess carbohydrates, not fat, that causes weight gain, low-carb proponents advocate restricting carbohydrate intake to as little as 20 grams per day or less, depending on the plan. According to the Food and Nutrition Board of the Institute of Medicine of the National Academies of Science, the recommended daily allowance of carbohydrates for children between ages one and eighteen is a minimum of 100 grams.

As of early 2004, both Atkins Nutritionals and Dr. Barry Sears (creator of "The Zone") stated that they do not recommend their plans for children and only market their related diet products to adults. However, Dr. Arthur Agatston, the author of *The South Beach Diet*, does recommend his plan for children, as long as they omit the two-week introductory phase of the program. The same goes for Drs. Michael and Mary Dan Eades, Protein Power creators, who say that their program can be used for children as long as they start with Phase II. SugarBusters, which is less restrictive than Atkins in terms of carbohydrate allowances, has a specific plan geared towards children.

How It Works

The carbohydrates your child consumes in food are the main power source for cellular energy and central nervous system functioning. Carbs convert to glucose, and the pancreas pumps out insulin that "unlocks" cells and allows the glucose energy inside. Low-carb proponents say that consuming too many carbs overloads this finely balanced system and triggers the release of too much insulin, which is eventually stored as excess fat. Excess circulating insulin is also associated with insulin resistance and raises heart disease risk.

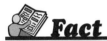 **Fact**

A 2003 study at Johns Hopkins found that children following a low-carb/low-protein/high-fat ketogenic diet (which has been found effective for seizure control in children with epilepsy) ended up with dramatically higher cholesterol levels after six months on the diet. Note that unlike most low-carb plans, the ketogenic diet is purposefully low in protein, so it is unclear whether these results would translate to other low-carb plans studied in children.

When dietary carbs are reduced, the body turns to the only other source of energy available for fuel—body fat. This process of burning fat for energy is known as ketosis. It can result in weight loss, although ketosis may also have some undesirable side-effects including bad breath, headaches, nausea, fatigue, and dehydration if fluid intake isn't increased. Low-carb plans usually focus on increasing dietary protein as well, which is known to promote satiety (or feelings of fullness).

Atkins and other low-carb plans replace sugars and starches with protein-rich foods, such as red meat and eggs. Critics of carb-reduction say that the high levels of artery-clogging fats and cholesterol from foods like this are a one-way ticket to heart disease. Interestingly, several studies have concluded that after six and twelve months, individuals on a reduced carbohydrate diet actually improved their blood cholesterol profiles. But there are no long-term (longer than one year) studies that measure the impact of low-carb/high-protein eating on the cardiovascular system, so the jury is still out.

Kids and Carbs

While studies have shown that low-carb eating does indeed promote faster weight loss than low-fat plans, studies specific to children, as well as long-term adult studies, are sorely lacking. And the fact is that any dietary plan that excludes or dramatically slashes a wide variety of nutrient-filled foods is not good for your child. Kids need carbs—for energy, for brain development and cognitive function, and for overall growth. The introductory phases of diet plans like Atkins and South Beach cut out or greatly restrict essential foods that kids need for nutrients, including milk and some other dairy, some fruits and veggies, and many grains (including pasta, breads, and cereals).

Is cutting your child's overall daily carb intake a bad idea? Remember the golden rule of weight management—that calories are what count. If your child is getting a lot of extra calories in the form of too many refined carbohydrates (such as from chips, fries, donuts, or sugary drinks and cereals), it makes sense to cut back. Even if those foods were not high in carbs, they aren't nutrient dense and therefore aren't great choices to begin with. Choose those carbs that have some redeeming nutritional value—like veggies, fruits, whole-wheat breads, and whole-grain pastas and cereals.

As always, speak with your child's doctor and a registered dietitian if you are interested in following a more formal program of carbohydrate reduction for your family.

Popular low-carb and reduced-carb diet plans include the following:

- **Atkins.** The granddaddy of all the low-carb plans, Atkins advocates an initial "induction phase," in which daily carb consumption is 20 grams or less, and ultimately ends in "lifetime maintenance," with a daily carb allowance between 25 and 90 grams.

- **Protein Power.** Similar to Atkins, Protein Power is a three-phase program that starts with a maximum of 30 daily grams of carbs and gradually increases carbohydrates to a "maintenance level."
- **South Beach.** Emphasizes carbohydrate quality over quantity, encouraging a variety of low-glycemic carbohydrates.
- **SugarBusters.** The only one of the reduced-carb plans that has a program geared towards children, SugarBusters recommends that kids have a daily mix of 50 percent carbs (primarily from high-fiber sources), 30 percent fat, and 20 percent protein. It also focuses on reducing sugar in the diet.
- **The Zone.** Being in "The Zone" refers to keeping insulin levels in balance through a low-glycemic load diet that derives 35 to 45 percent of daily calories from carbohydrates (based on an 1,100 or 1,400 calorie daily diet for women and men, respectively).

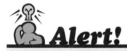

Alert!

People with existing kidney impairment, or those who are at risk for kidney disease, should never attempt a high-protein diet plan. Low-carb, high-protein diets also pose a risk of kidney stones (due to elevated levels of uric acid in the bloodstream) and a loss of bone mass (due to insufficient calcium intake). The high levels of saturated fat that can accompany these diets may also promote high cholesterol and heart problems, although clinical studies have yet to demonstrate a positive association between the two.

The Glycemic Index

The last three of these plans—SugarBusters, South Beach, and The Zone—are based on the concept of choosing the "right" types of carbohydrates, those with a low glycemic index and/or glycemic load. (SugarBusters calls it "insulin response.") The glycemic index is a measurement of how quickly the carbohydrates in specific foods raise blood sugar levels (and subsequently, insulin levels) on a scale of 0 to 100. Foods with a high glycemic index (over 70), or GI ranking, will trigger a quick spike in blood glucose levels, while low-GI foods (under 55) cause a slow and steady rise.

The GI has several limitations. First of all, not all foods have a glycemic index rating. The laboratory procedure for assessing the GI of a food is time-consuming and expensive, and only a few facilities in the world have the proper equipment and protocols in place to do the testing correctly. Second, the GI by itself doesn't give you the whole picture. Some foods may have a high GI but contain relatively little carbohydrate to begin with. A second tool, known as the glycemic load (GL), is a measurement of the GI of a food multiplied by the grams of available carbohydrate (carbohydrate minus fiber content) found in one serving. A GL of ten or less is considered low.

While the concepts of glycemic load and glycemic index can be helpful in food selection and are extremely useful for individuals trying to establish dietary control of diabetes, they are probably way too complex for your child to use on a daily basis. In fact, they can even be overly complicated for the math-challenged adult. Learning more about those whole foods that provide the best nutritional bang for the buck is probably a better use of your time and effort. Generally speaking, whole unrefined and unprocessed foods that are high in fiber, such as broccoli, strawberries, and whole-grain cereals, will have a low GL anyway.

Low-Fat Diets: The Facts

Since the late 1970s, when Dr. Nathan Pritikin introduced his low-fat focused Pritikin Program for Diet and Exercise, fat has been the dietary enemy in the battle of the bulge. There are a number of clinically proven reasons to cut the fat out of your family's diet. Too much dietary fat, particularly saturated fat, can raise your risk for heart disease, stroke, and some cancers.

Drastic reduction or elimination of fat from the diet is not recommended and can even be dangerous for children. Kids need some dietary fat for energy, growth, and development; to absorb fat-soluble vitamins such as A, D, E, and K; and to keep skin and hair healthy. They also need the essential fatty acids found in fatty coldwater fish, some oils, and soybeans. Restricting fat before a child turns two could have an impact on the developing brain and central nervous system. The American Academy of Pediatrics recommends that children over age two eat no less than 20 percent and no more than 30 percent of their total daily calories from fat.

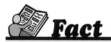 **Fact**

Omega-3 fatty acids, found in coldwater fish, flaxseed, walnuts, wheat germ, and soybeans, are important nutrients for heart health and disease prevention. They are also critical for brain and visual development in children.

In the end, it's calories that count. And gram-for-gram, fat has more calories than both protein and carbohydrates (9 per gram for fat versus 4 per gram for carbs and protein). So lowering fat can make a big difference in your child's daily diet.

But that doesn't mean you should go overboard on low-fat and reduced-fat food products. Many replace fat with added sugar, and added calories. And sometimes people perceive the low-fat label as a license to overindulge, eating much more than they would if it were a "full-fat" version. Trim excess fat naturally—by choosing foods that are intrinsically lower in saturated fats.

Food Franchises

Most center-based weight-loss programs are adult-oriented, but some may accommodate children. Yet some of the reasons these programs work—accountability through meeting attendance, group motivation, weekly weigh-ins—may not always be a successful approach for children.

Weight Watchers

Weight Watchers—perhaps the most recognized weight-loss program in the United States—was founded in the early 1960s. The program is designed around weekly peer and leader meetings that provide support, education, and a sense of accountability. The current program uses a points system that assigns a point value to certain foods. Based on current weight, goal weight, and activity level, Weight Watchers members are allotted a certain number of points that they can consume each day.

The program does allow children between the ages of ten and sixteen to participate at many meeting locations, provided that they have a signed doctor's note that indicates their weight goal, and a signed health release form from their parents.

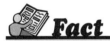 **Fact**

A 2004 study found that among people who completed both the weight loss and the maintenance phases of the Weight Watchers program, participants reported maintaining up to 87 percent of their weight loss after two years had passed, and over half their weight loss at the five-year mark.

Other Weight Loss Programs

There are a handful of formal programs that have been developed specifically for children. One of these—Shapedown—was developed in 1979 at the University of California School of Medicine, San Francisco.

Shapedown is a ten-week, age-appropriate program designed for children, adolescents, and their parents that incorporates weekly support groups, food and activity journals, and workbooks with a focus on family lifestyle changes towards fitness. The program is usually based in community hospitals and health-care facilities, and group instructors (who are typically health-care professionals) undergo a minimum of forty-six hours of clinical education and training in the program from the University of California. A study published in the *Journal of the American Dietetic Association* found that kids who participated in the program achieved long-term (fifteen month) relative weight loss and had improved self-esteem and nutrition and fitness knowledge. See Appendix B for contact information for Shapedown.

Weight loss or fitness camps can be an additional source of assistance in the quest for weight control for some families. When looking at camps, make sure you choose one that is both accredited by the American Camping Association and that incorporates family education into its program. Chapter 13 has more information on camps.

Nutritional Counseling

Unless you're a fairly decent musician yourself, you wouldn't try to teach your child how to play the piano without a piano instructor. You might get as far as teaching her to plunk out *Mary Had a Little Lamb,* but the finer points that are the foundation for a good pianist, like reading music and proper hand position, would be lost. Similarly, many parents think that they can revamp their child's dietary habits with a few new recipes or the latest popular diet. Taking the time to see a professional, in this case a registered dietitian (RD), will be invaluable in providing you and your child with the underlying skills you need to eat healthy for life.

An RD offers you the following services:

- **Customized care.** A registered dietitian will look at your child's particular medical and lifestyle needs and design a dietary plan just for her.
- **Ready reference.** Most RDs are happy to take follow-up phone

calls after your initial appointment to help with your questions and concerns.

- **Experience.** Registered dietitians have completed at least a bachelor's degree in nutrition, have finished a long-term supervised professional practice program, and have passed a rigorous national examination to earn the RD designation.
- **Specialization.** An RD with a CSP designation is a board-certified specialist in pediatric nutrition who has passed a comprehensive examination and has at least 4,000 hours of recent (in the past five years) practical experience in a pediatric setting.
- **The latest and greatest.** In order to maintain the RD designation, registered dietitians must continue to take professional education coursework each year throughout their careers, keeping them at the forefront of nutrition knowledge.

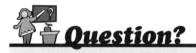

Question?

What's the difference between a registered dietitian and a DTR?
DTR stands for "dietetic technician, registered." A DTR has completed a minimum of a two-year associate's degree in a dietetics technology program from an accredited U.S. college or university, has supervised practical experience in the dietetic field, and has passed a national examination. An RD (registered dietitian) has a four-year bachelor's degree and more extensive field practice. Either can probably provide you with a useful consultation if the individual has adequate experience with pediatric patients.

What to Expect

When booking an appointment, ask if the RD would like a copy of your child's medical record sent over from your child's primary care provider before the initial appointment. The RD will need to obtain a detailed medical history during your child's nutritional assessment, and having her file on hand can be helpful.

The initial visit is usually a nutritional assessment, during which the dietitian will ask questions about your child's (and your family's) lifestyle and eating habits and health history. You'll discuss any food allergies or intolerances; religious beliefs and cultural or ethnic background that may affect your family's dietary intake; and your child's food likes and dislikes. You may also talk about your overall health and nutrition goals. Once the RD has all the necessary background information, she'll develop a nutritional plan customized to your child's (and your family's) needs. This may be at the initial visit, or it may be at a follow-up appointment.

 Essential

In the United States, dietitians are regulated and licensed at the state level. The designation "LD" indicates a dietician has a license to practice. Remember that a nutritionist is not the same thing as a DTR or RD. Nutritionists are not professionally regulated, and there are no educational, experience, or licensing requirements to use the title of nutritionist.

Dietary education is also part of an RD's job. During your initial appointment, or at a follow-up session, you will receive printed information and/or verbal instructions on the food pyramid, reading nutritional labels, daily caloric goals, vitamins and minerals, portion sizes, and more. She may also provide sample menus and recipes for your use. The number of sessions you'll need with the RD will vary. She may recommend periodic follow-up appointments to assess how your child and family are progressing. Or you may find that one intensive session, with the opportunity for follow-up phone calls, is enough.

No Quick-Fix Solutions

Diets appeal to the American need for instant, or at least short-term, gratification. Unfortunately, there are no quick and easy solutions to a weight problem. While you can gain some insight from some popular diet programs—such as cutting out sugar, à la Atkins, and reducing saturated fat as Pritikin prescribes—only a fundamental change in the way your family approaches food and exercise will make the difference.

Stay focused on the idea that you're in this for the long haul and that you are giving your child the skills he needs to continue this new way of healthy eating as he grows into adulthood. Remember that daily exercise is an absolutely essential part of not just weight loss but overall fitness. Getting that before-breakfast walk or after-dinner bike ride in is just as important as what you have to eat for breakfast and dinner.

Chapter 8

Food for Thought: Helping Kids Eat Intelligently

How do you help your children make good dietary choices? Arm them with knowledge about their nutritional requirements, involve them in the process of menu planning and meal preparation, and teach them to recognize and respond to their own feelings of hunger and fullness. You also need to educate them about what foods are off-limits, and why, while at the same time providing healthy and kid-friendly taste alternatives.

The Benefits of Breastfeeding

Choosing to breastfeed your child will start her off on the right path nutritionally. Breast milk is the perfect nutrient match for your infant, and some clinical studies have found that infants who are breastfed are less likely to have weight problems in childhood. The "feed on demand" system that breastfeeding promotes can help both you and your baby become more attuned to her natural hunger and satiety cues.

That said, not everyone chooses to breastfeed. Sometimes maternal or infant medical conditions prevent lactation or latching. In other cases, career or other logistical concerns make formula-feeding a better choice for your family. You should know that even if you breastfeed for a short period, such as during your maternity leave, it can be beneficial for your child.

If you do formula-feed your baby, follow her natural hunger cues and don't attempt to impose an artificial schedule on her. It won't work, and you'll both be frustrated with the result. You also want to teach her early on that her hunger and fullness cues have value and should regulate her feedings.

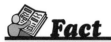 **Fact**

> If you're breastfeeding, the American Dietetic Association recommends that you follow the food pyramid, and add an extra serving from each food group each day. You should also drink plenty of fluids to prevent dehydration. You can be sure that your baby is getting enough to eat if she is making six or more wet and two or three dirty diapers daily and is also gaining weight.

Building an Informed Consumer

Getting your family on the right track nutritionally requires an education in nutrition basics, the difference between marketing messages and nutrition facts, daily dietary requirements, and how to decipher food labels.

Virtually everyone can benefit from a visit to a registered dietitian, or RD. An RD can look at your current meal and eating patterns and suggest changes for improvement. Taking a food log into the RD's office is often helpful. It's a good idea to make an appointment for the entire family to attend to keep your child from feeling singled out and so that he feels supported in the group effort to improve family nutrition.

Your child's pediatrician should be able to provide a referral to a registered dietitian who has experience working with children and families. The American Dietetic Association can also help you find an RD in your area. See Appendix B for contact information.

Teaching Your Child About Food Labels

You will find the nutrition facts label on virtually every packaged food product in your local grocery store. It can be a wealth of information—if you know how to read it correctly. Although total grams and milligrams of certain nutrients are listed, the most revealing information on the nutritional facts is the daily value, or DV. Daily values (or DV) are expressed as a percentage of the maximum recommended dietary allowance for the day, based on an "average" 2,000-calorie diet. For example, if a food's sodium content represents 50 percent of the daily value, and your child eats one serving of the product, he will have consumed half of his sodium allowance for the entire day.

Serving Sizes and Calories

The first entry on the food label is serving size and number of servings per package. Teach your child to assess the serving size in relationship to how much she typically eats of the food. For example, if she eats two servings of a food, she should double the nutritional percentages and values on the package.

After servings is a listing of total calories and calories from fat per serving. You and your child should assess this information in the context of her daily calorie needs for the day. Chapter 5 provides more information on recommended daily caloric intake.

Nutrients to Limit

Nutrients that should be limited—fat, cholesterol, sodium, carbohydrates, and protein—are next. Both total grams and daily values are included. Trans fats are also included on some labels and should be limited as well (see "The Trouble with Trans Fats," below). Again, the DV is a good indicator of how much of a particular nutrient your child will get from a food. Levels of 20 percent or higher for any of these dietary elements are considered high. Teach your child to compare product labels of different brands to make healthier food choices.

Total carbohydrates are the next item on the food label, and these are also listed in total grams and as a percentage of daily value. Two subcategories—dietary fiber and sugars—are listed individually under the total carbohydrates. Generally speaking, look for foods with high fiber content and low sugar content. Protein rounds out the list of primary nutrients included on the food label.

Vitamins and Minerals

Next come the vitamins and minerals that you want to ensure your child gets plenty of—vitamin A, vitamin C, calcium, and iron. Your child should learn that his food choices throughout the day should total 100 percent of the daily value for these nutrients.

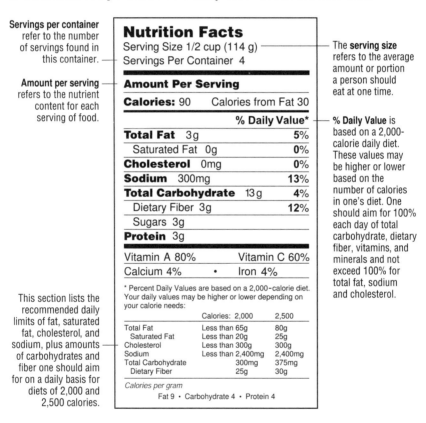

Servings per container refer to the number of servings found in this container.

Amount per serving refers to the nutrient content for each serving of food.

The **serving size** refers to the average amount or portion a person should eat at one time.

% Daily Value is based on a 2,000-calorie daily diet. These values may be higher or lower based on the number of calories in one's diet. One should aim for 100% each day of total carbohydrate, dietary fiber, vitamins, and minerals and not exceed 100% for total fat, sodium and cholesterol.

This section lists the recommended daily limits of fat, saturated fat, cholesterol, and sodium, plus amounts of carbohydrates and fiber one should aim for on a daily basis for diets of 2,000 and 2,500 calories.

Nutrition Facts

Serving Size 1/2 cup (114 g)
Servings Per Container 4

Amount Per Serving

Calories: 90   Calories from Fat 30

                                            % Daily Value*

Total Fat 3g	5%
Saturated Fat 0g	0%
Cholesterol 0mg	0%
Sodium 300mg	13%
Total Carbohydrate 13 g	4%
Dietary Fiber 3g	12%
Sugars 3g	
Protein 3g	

Vitamin A 80%	Vitamin C 60%
Calcium 4% •	Iron 4%

* Percent Daily Values are based on a 2,000-calorie diet. Your daily values may be higher or lower depending on your calorie needs:

	Calories: 2,000	2,500
Total Fat	Less than 65g	80g
Saturated Fat	Less than 20g	25g
Cholesterol	Less than 300g	300g
Sodium	Less than 2,400mg	2,400mg
Total Carbohydrate	300mg	375mg
Dietary Fiber	25g	30g

Calories per gram
Fat 9 • Carbohydrate 4 • Protein 4

FIGURE 9-1: Nutrition Food Label.

Quick Reference

To provide a convenient frame of reference, the footnote located at the bottom of the nutrition facts panel includes all total daily values (in grams) for the main nutrients included on the label (fat, saturated fat, cholesterol, sodium, carbohydrates, fiber) based on a diet of 2,000 calories per day. On larger packages there is also a list of total daily values for a 2,500-calorie diet. Remember that your child's caloric needs will vary based on age and gender.

Unlabeled Items

There are cases in which food won't be labeled, and a good nutrition guidebook will come in handy. Foods that don't require labeling under FDA and USDA guidelines include these items:

- Foods sold for immediate consumption (including food from vendors, restaurant meals, and airplane food)
- Food prepared "on-site" for later consumption (such as products from a bakery)
- Foods manufactured or prepared by certain small businesses that do not exceed prescribed employee and production guidelines and who have filed an exemption with the FDA
- Foods shipped in bulk, like produce

Nights at the Round Table

When was the last time your whole family sat down together for a leisurely evening meal with no interruptions or distractions? Aside from being a great opportunity to share your day and keep in touch with what's going on in each other's lives, meals together are a golden opportunity for you to get healthy food options in front of your child.

Making Meals Family Time

Placing a priority on meals eaten together also shows your child that you value time spent together. As children grow older, their extracurricular activities can cut into family meals, as can a hectic work schedule and other commitments for adults. Try to remain flexible in your quest for family meals. Make dinner earlier or later to accommodate family members, as necessary. When meals are moved later, make sure you have healthy snacks (raw veggies and dip, fruit slices) on hand to keep hungry kids happy while they wait. When family schedules make regular dinners together logistically impossible, then try focusing on breakfast instead. It may mean getting up an extra half-hour or hour early and getting your child into the early-rising routine as well, but the benefits gained are well worth it. For children who traditionally haven't been big breakfast eaters or who rely on prepackaged grab-and-go breakfast snacks, instituting a family breakfast is an excellent way to replace bad habits with healthy new ones.

Getting Kids into the Cooking Act

Cooking with your kids can get them more excited about family meals and about healthy foods in general. A self-professed veggie-hater who gets the opportunity to clean and cook her own can rarely resist at least trying the final result. You may find a more adventurous eater on your hands as you allow your children to play a part in choosing recipes, shopping for ingredients, and preparing foods.

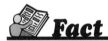 **Fact**

Beyond being an opportunity to learn about healthful foods, cooking with you can benefit your kids in other ways. Reading a recipe requires the ability to comprehend and follow directions, measuring ingredients sharpens math skills, activities like adding yeast to dough involves science, and of course making a mess is always fun.

As your children grow older, they may be less excited by the prospect of helping mom stir ingredients or setting the table. Move them up a level to menu planning—let them select recipes and even prepare a meal solo (or with you, under their direction). It's also a great way to teach them how to plan a well-balanced meal.

The Right Atmosphere

Retire the TV trays, and the television, at dinnertime. Conversation among family members should provide sufficient entertainment. If the phone rings during dinner, let your answering machine or voice mail pick it up. Better yet, turn off the ringer. Same goes for cell phones, beepers (unless you're on call for a heart transplant), and any other communications devices. Don't read the paper, work on your laptop, program your PDA, or introduce any other distraction to mealtime. Consider the family dinner the same as an important meal with a client or a first date. You wouldn't ignore your fellow diner in that situation, so keep your focus on your family and enjoying a healthy meal together.

Kitchen Tools

Once you have your kids on board for cooking, make sure you have the tools to get the job done right. That goes for everything from food to cooking utensils. If your experience in the kitchen has been limited up until now, you might explore taking a cooking class at your local community college or even investing in some basic general-interest how-to type cookbooks. You can also explore the resources listed in Appendix B in the back of this book for cooking and meal-planning information.

A good set of measuring tools for cooking and baking is essential. If they aren't in your kitchen already, purchase both liquid and dry measuring cups and spoons. Also important is an accurate gram and/or ounce scale for measuring portion sizes. Why measure? If you've fallen into the habit of dishing out heaping double portions, a scale can get you back on track. You may be surprised at how much a single serving really is once you start measuring.

By teaching your child how to accurately weigh portion sizes, she can learn to estimate servings more accurately while she's away from home. For example, three ounces of meat or poultry is similar in dimension to a deck of cards, while an ounce of cheese is about the size of an AA battery.

Always shop with a grocery list. Going in with no definite ideas of what you're going to purchase, particularly when you're hungry, can be an expensive and unhealthy proposition. Impulse buys can lead to extra fat, sugar, and cholesterol in your cart—and once it's purchased, you'll have a harder time just saying no.

The Hit List

While emphasizing moderation is the most practical and successful approach to limiting sweets and fats in your child's diet, there are some calorie-dense foods and beverages that simply have no redeeming nutritional value. These should be severely limited, if not cut out completely from your family meal plan.

The Trouble with Trans Fats

Trans fats, or trans fatty acids, are identifiable by the words "hydrogenated" or "partially hydrogenated" fat on a food label. They are artery-clogging, nonpliable fats that are associated with high total and LDL (bad) cholesterol, low HDL (good) cholesterol, cardiovascular disease, diabetes, obesity, and other chronic health problems. They're often added to processed foods because of their preservative qualities. These are actually unsaturated vegetable-based fats that are put through a process known as hydrogenation to stabilize them.

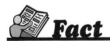 **Fact**

Based on a 2,000 calorie diet, total daily fat intake should not exceed 65 grams according to USDA recommendations. Of those 65 grams, the combined level of saturated and/or trans fats should not be more than 20 grams.

Foods that are frequently high in trans fats include stick margarines, packaged high-fat donuts and baked goods, vegetable shortening, fried foods, and many potato and corn chips. In 2003, the FDA enacted new regulatory guidelines that will require food manufacturers to include trans-fat content information on nutrition facts labeling by 2006. Some manufacturers have complied early, and you can find trans-fat information listed on some packaged goods already.

The Hard Truth on Soft Drinks

So-called soft drinks—soda pop, sports beverages, fruit-flavored drink mixes—are stuffed with added sugars, calories, and caffeine. They aren't a significant source of any nutrient that helps build strong bodies. The USDA reports that soft drinks are the number-one source of added (refined) sugars in the processed food chain. Although exact sugar content varies by brand and type, on average a 12-ounce can of soda contains right around 40 grams (or ten teaspoons) of sugar.

According to the National Soft Drink Association, in 2002, the average American consumed almost 53 gallons of soft drinks (over a gallon a week). Even juice-based drinks can be a problem. Many drinks you may assume are primarily fruit juice are full of added sugars and contain little, if any, real fruit juice. Always check the nutrition facts label to find out how much added sugar is in your child's beverage of choice.

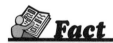 **Fact**

A 2001 study published in *The Lancet* found that among subjects aged eleven and twelve, each additional sugar-sweetened drink per day they consumed raised both their BMI and their obesity risk, independent of the foods they ate and the amount of physical activity they got.

Water is always a good choice for thirst quenching, but it can get old fast for kids who were formerly hooked on carbonated sodas. There are many fruit-flavored bottled waters now on the market—both with carbonation and without—that your child may find satisfying. If your child is a die-hard soda junkie, try switching him to a diet version that uses an artificial sweetener instead of refined sugars.

Sensible Snacks

So now that you've helped your child recognize what not to eat, how about providing some good alternatives for those after-school snacks? Consider your child's tastes when suggesting nutritious yet tasty and appealing snack foods. Try to make choices that are high in fiber and protein and low in fat. If she's a French fry fanatic, try substituting baked sweet-potato wedges. Chocolate peanut-butter cup fans may go for sliced fresh fruit topped with a dollop of peanut butter. Here are a few more sensible snack ideas:

- If they like jellied "fruit" snacks, try raisins or dehydrated fruit mixes—but check the label for added sugars.
- If they like chips and onion dip, try raw veggie sticks and low-fat ranch dressing, or low-fat popcorn.
- If they like cheese curls or fat-filled cheese crackers, try low-fat cheese sticks.
- If they like Popsicles, try 100 percent frozen fruit juice bars or frozen fresh fruits.
- If they like ice cream, try low-fat fruit-flavored yogurt in frozen or unfrozen varieties.

Get creative, and don't be afraid to try new ideas. Buying in small quantities will ensure minimum waste if the snack is a dud. Let your kids brainstorm new noshing choices, and involve them in the mixing, slicing, and dicing when appropriate. Chances are your child will like the healthier choices just as much, if not more, than the high-fat, high-sugar original.

Satiety Strategies

Satiety, or the feeling of fullness you get after a meal, is what triggers the stomach to send the "Stop eating!" signal to the brain. The biological processes that control this process involve the hypothalamus (the hormone regulatory center of the brain), as well as certain gut hormones, changes in the digestive tract, and blood glucose levels. It takes approximately twenty minutes from the start of a meal for these complex processes to occur and for the brain to receive and recognize the satiety signal. This time lag is why people who gulp down meals often overeat—they aren't giving their body sufficient time to let them know they're full.

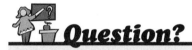 **Question?**

What's the satiety index?
The satiety index (or SI) is a scale that rates foods on their ability to generate a feeling of fullness. It was developed by researchers at the University of Sydney, who created the index by feeding 240-calorie portions of various foods to study subjects and then assessing their perceived satiety and follow-up eating behaviors. Donuts have a relatively low SI of 68 percent, while boiled potatoes, porridge, and oranges rank among the highest on the index.

To discourage overeating past a feeling of fullness, keep these strategies for satiety in mind:

- **It's not a race.** Ask your child not to rush through meals or finish sandwiches in three bites. See if you can prolong the actual time at mealtime that is spent eating to round out at about twenty minutes, the magic number for satiety.
- **Pack in the protein.** In general, protein-rich foods have a high satiety index (as well as being beneficial for developing bodies), so try to include a protein punch in each meal.

- **Bulk up.** Fibrous foods delay stomach emptying. Thus, they can make you feel fuller faster and longer, as well as providing other health benefits.
- **Don't skip meals.** If your child sits down to the table ravenous, she's more likely to eat too quickly and eat past hunger.
- **Encourage appetizers.** When she's really hungry, suggest a nutritious snack of fruit or raw veggies twenty minutes before mealtime to take the edge off her appetite.

Above all, encourage your child to listen to her body and trust the signals that it sends her. Ignoring her hunger can be just as detrimental as ignoring satiety.

CHAPTER 9

Meals on Wheels: Eating Out Sensibly

O n average, Americans spend almost half of their food dollars eating outside the home. And with over 875 billion restaurants in the United States, there are plenty of choices available. While eating out can be fun and convenient, it's also fraught with potential pitfalls for your family—such as huge portions, fat-laden fare, and kids' menus packed with empty calories. Don't confine yourself to the kitchen just yet, however. With planning and a little cooperation from your favorite restaurants, dining out can still be part of your family's lifestyle.

Driving Past the Drive-Through

Every parent succumbs to the quick and easy allure of the drive-through lane for lunch or dinner once in a while. It seems so easy to pick up a couple of Happy Meals for the kids to scarf down on the way to wherever the family is headed and shave a few minutes off your time-starved schedule. Sometimes the kids badger you into it, having just seen the fast-food commercial for the latest toy, "available for a limited time only" and a requirement with their meal.

Eating on the run means you and your children aren't practicing mindful eating. You aren't enjoying your meal, nor are you eating it with a presence of mind. It takes the social aspect out of the family meal, too—driving with a steering wheel in one hand and a burger in the other doesn't leave much additional attention for conversation.

And then there's the food. Fast-food restaurants are not known for their healthy menu options, and when they are available, items such as salads aren't really built for four-wheel-dining.

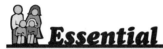 **Essential**

> While drive-through visits that promote grab-and-go eating aren't ideal, that's doesn't mean you have to forsake all modern conveniences. In the dead of winter or driving rain, by all means use the drive-through. Just make it a rule that all food and drink stays in the bag until you're home and seated around the family table together. This also gives you the opportunity to order salads, soups, and other menu items that aren't well suited for dashboard dining.

How Fast Food Promotes Fat Kids

So what's so bad about fast food, anyway? Take the cooking methods, for starters. Deep-frying is king at many fast-food establishments. This method cooks quickly and evenly and allows restaurant chains to produce standardized food products. When cooking oil is hydrogenated, that means your child is also getting a large order of unhealthy, artery-clogging trans fats in the bargain. Fast food also tends to be highly processed, low in fiber, and high in sodium.

A cheeseburger, small order of fries, and small (12-ounce) chocolate shake at McDonald's will net your child a whopping 990 calories and 37 grams of fat (16 grams of it saturated, 81 percent of the RDA), according to the restaurant's nutritional facts. Increase that to large fries and a double cheeseburger with a small shake, and you've reached 1,440 calories and 64 grams of fat. That's 98 percent of your child's daily allotment, with 25 grams of the total being saturated fat, equivalent to 123 percent of the daily RDA. And that's just one meal of the day.

Burger franchises are far and away the most popular fast-food destinations in the United States, with the four largest chains raking in over $40 billion in sales in 2002. Of course there are other options beyond burgers and fries in fast food. Just about any cuisine has a fast food purveyor these days. Good strategies for choosing among them wisely include the following:

- **Burgers.** If whole-bran buns are available, opt for one. Don't super-size those fries; if you can talk your child into a garden side salad instead, that's even better.
- **Chicken.** Grilled or rotisserie-style chicken is a better choice than anything deep-fried. It's also smart to skip the gravy. Some chicken places offer a wide variety of side dishes. Avoid salads and sides swimming in sauce, and go for the vegetables instead.
- **Seafood.** If you can find anything not covered in batter and deep-fried, order it. Breading soaks up the grease and adds more fat to the food. If not, you'd do better to order as small a portion as possible or steer clear completely.
- **Subs and sandwiches.** Choose whole-grain breads, low-fat dressings, and lots of veggie toppings. Keep sandwiches a reasonable size, and try fresh fruits or vegetable-based salads for sides.
- **Soups and salads.** Probably the healthiest options, but there are still some potential pitfalls. Avoid rich cream-based soups, if possible; keep it to a cup if not. Be selective about salad toppings. A salad topped with fried chicken and extra cheese and dressing can be just as full of fat and calories as a burger-and-fries combo.
- **Donuts and bagels.** Make donuts a rare indulgence. Bagels (particularly whole-grain ones) are a better choice, in moderation. Choose low-fat cream cheeses and sugar-free jams as spreads.
- **Mexican, Italian, and Asian.** The key to remember is to keep portions under control. Don't order a bigger pizza than your

family can handle, and don't frequent all-you-can-eat Chinese buffets. More cuisine-specific tips on ethnic foods are offered throughout the rest of this chapter.

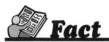 *Fact*

According to the National Restaurant Association, Americans spent $2,276 per household, or $910 per person, on dining out in 2002. Takeout and delivery accounts for over half of all U.S. restaurant business.

Making Better Fast-Food Choices

It's tough to try and sell your child on a grilled chicken sandwich and a salad when the hamburger and fries combo comes with the latest kid's movie character or the cool toy of the week. Marketing to kids is the name of the game in many fast-food establishments, and that can be a powerful influence for parents to try and combat. Adding a prize to a box of deep-fried food sends the underlying message that fatty foods are fun and rewarding.

When your kids are younger, the best strategy is often simply to avoid places where high-fat, high-calorie kids' meals are marketed with toys. It's hard to make your message about healthy foods stick when you're competing with Beanie Babies or the latest Disney movie characters. But if you must go, and you feel you absolutely must get the toy—for example, if you're dining with another family and their child has ordered a meal with a prize—some establishments will sell it separately at a nominal fee upon request. Don't be shy about letting the manager, and the corporate headquarters of the restaurant franchise, know your feelings about offering this little "reward" with healthier menu choices, too.

Restaurant chains are becoming more aware of special dietary needs and health-consciousness of their patrons and are making nutritional information more readily available to customers. Some are also adding more health-conscious selections—such as salads, grilled chicken sandwiches, and sandwich wraps—to their menus. Ask the places you frequent for a copy of their nutritional analysis of menu items, or look for the information online (see Appendix B for resources). If they don't have them available, once again let the manager know you'd like to see them in the future; like most retail businesses, consumer demand is what drives change in the food service industry.

Finally, as in all things, moderation is important. As your child grows older, she'll be visiting the places her friends visit, and fast-food hangouts will likely be among them. To say "no thanks" when everyone else is indulging is hard and may be an unrealistic expectation for you to have of your child. An occasional fast-food burger and (small) order of fries isn't the end of the world, as long as it doesn't become a regular habit and your child recognizes it as the exception rather than the norm.

The Best—and Worst—Restaurant Choices

Sit-down restaurants, whether casual-dining or upscale establishments, offer a bit more flexibility for your family than the cookie-cutter offerings of fast-food franchises. Menu items can often be cooked to your specifications, and it's easier to get answers about how dishes are prepared and what ingredients are used. Knowing what to look for in advance can help you help your child order more healthily.

A key question to ask is what type of oil foods are cooked in. Those prepared in 100-percent polyunsaturated and monounsaturated oils (such as olive, canola, corn, safflower, soybean, and peanut) are best. Lard, animal fats, partially hydrogenated vegetable oils, and tropical oils (palm and coconut) should be avoided if at all possible. The good news is that no matter what your family's favorite style of food, there's bound to be something on the menu that your child can enjoy. Following are the best and worst on the table for four popular ethnic cuisine types.

Chinese and Other Asian

This cuisine has plenty going for it. Asian food is high in vegetables and often steamed or stir-fried. Stir-fry is usually cooked in healthier oils such as sesame or peanut oil. Unless you're eating at a buffet or fast-food establishment, food is typically cooked to order, meaning you can make healthy substitutions and requests (such as sautéing or steaming instead of frying). Finally, family style serving means that you and your child can share a few dishes and not feel pressured into eating huge portions. Use the chopsticks and you all may eat even less!

Among the cons to the Chinese menu is the tendency to deep-frying. Selections are often predominantly deep-fried delicacies, such as egg rolls, wontons, and fried poultry dishes (among Japanese foods, tempura and fried dumplings are the dishes to avoid). Sauces can be calorie-, sugar-, and sodium-laden, so order them on the side or pass altogether. Fried rice is also filled with extra fat, so opt for the steamed white variety instead.

Mexican

Mexican food gives you plenty of reasons to say "Olé!" Salsa (green or red) and pico de gallo are great low-fat sauces that spice up just about anything on the table. Salads are usually available at most Mexican restaurants; just make sure they serve your child's in a bowl instead of a deep-fried tortilla shell, and leave off the sour cream and guacamole. Other good choices are chicken fajitas, soft chicken tacos, and chicken or beef enchiladas and burritos. Cheese is often used liberally on some of these items, and since that can add a lot of fat to the dish, ask that it be light or served on the side.

There are some factors on the con side as well. Many deep-fried menu items make Mexican food a potential pitfall for your child. Skip fried taco shells (go for the soft instead) as well as other fried items such as chimichangas, flautas, and sopapillas. Refried beans are often cooked with lard; if black beans are available, they're a good high-fiber choice. The unlimited supply of tortilla chips can make you feel stuffed before your order even hits the table. Either say "no thanks" to refills or skip them altogether. Other fat-filled ventures include guacamole, sour cream, and chili con queso (cheese dip). If you must have an appetizer, a warm soft tortilla (corn or flour) with zippy green or red salsa or pico de gallo is a better bet.

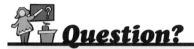

Question?

Is Japanese food healthy for our family?
Yes. Japanese food is one of the better choices available due to the low-fat cooking methods used in this cuisine (such as grilling, steaming, braising, broiling, and sautéing) and traditionally small portion sizes. Most dishes are heavy on the vegetables and low in added fat. Sushi and sashimi (thinly cut fresh fish) are very high in nutrients, but the uncooked fish poses a very real food safety risk. Cooked fish sushi is available at some restaurants, however; if your child is the adventuresome type, give it a try.

Italian

There's lots to love about Italian food. Pasta is low in fat, and it is available in many flavors (such as spinach, whole wheat, and tomato) as well as fun shapes and sizes. As for sauces, marinara and vegetable-based tomato sauces are delicious and low in calories. Stick with garden salads instead of potentially high-fat antipastos for a side dish. Pass on the veal (unless you know it's lean and prepared without breading) and prosciutto and go for grilled chicken or fish, both widely available as part of Italian dishes.

Italian food offers some pitfalls, though. Like chips in a Mexican restaurant, the bread basket can be your child's downfall when you eat Italian. Take a piece or two, then ask the server to take it away. Instead of butter or olive oil, ask for marinara sauce for dipping. (Olive oil isn't a bad option as long as it's used sparingly.) Skip the butter-soaked garlic bread and heavy cream sauces (like the ever-popular fettuccini alfredo), both heavy in fat, and hold the cheese (or at least go light). While pasta can be a good nutritional choice, watch the portion sizes. Helpings are often generous enough for two (or three).

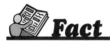 **Fact**

> Several pizza chains are offering lower-fat versions of the traditional pie. If your local pizza joint doesn't, you can cut the fat yourself by requesting half the cheese and all veggie toppings. Skip the stuffed crust, and opt for a thin version instead. Even better is a whole-wheat crust, if it's on the menu.

Middle Eastern

If you've never tried foods from the Middle East, now is a good time for an eating adventure. Nutrient-rich grains and legumes play a starring role in many Middle Eastern dishes such as tabouli, hummus, and couscous. Whole-grain pita pockets are a great alternative to bread and provide a nice accompaniment to dishes like hummus and tabouli. Middle Eastern foods are usually broiled, baked, grilled, or simmered, so added fat from frying is not a problem. shish kebab, which are typically offered in beef, lamb, or chicken varieties, are fun for kids to eat and are often served with skewered veggie chunks.

As with foods from anywhere in the world, there are things to look out for in Middle Eastern cuisine as well. Moussaka (fried eggplant in white sauce) and saganaki (fried cheese) are high in fat, as is tzatziki, the sauce that accompanies gyros. Sometimes tzatziki is prepared with yogurt instead of sour cream; when that's the case, it's a better choice so ask your server. Greek salads can be piled high with feta cheese, olives, and a liberal dose of high-calorie dressing, so ask for those items on the side if your child wants a salad.

Picking Family-Friendly Restaurants

A family-friendly restaurant consists of more than quick service, lids on the kids' cups, crayons and balloons, and a good supply of high chairs and booster seats. The menu should be amenable, or at least adaptable, to your family's health as well. Scout out good prospects in advance by talking to friends, reading reviews, and getting menu information with a phone call or through the company Web site when possible.

In cases where advance planning isn't possible, such as when you're on vacation or in an unfamiliar area, send an adult in to review the menu at the door before committing to a meal there. Even when you're out in the sticks and the corner diner is the only game in town, you still have some options for making it a family-friendly experience.

Customize the Cuisine

Don't be afraid to ask how foods are prepared, what cuts of meat are used, and what the serving sizes are in an effort to make the best choices for your family. If your child enjoys some of the healthier sides on the menu—maybe a garden salad, steamed vegetables, or fresh fruit—build a meal out of what's available. Any establishment that won't let you make reasonable requests for menu substitutions, like sauce on the side or steamed veggies instead of fries, doesn't want your business very much.

Portion Control

Americans like to get more for their money. In the case of restaurant food, this quest for value has clouded our nutritional vision. According to a 2002 study in the *American Journal of Public Health*, the average portion sizes in American restaurants and in other ready-to-eat marketplace foods have crept up steadily since the 1970s. Serving sizes virtually always exceed USDA recommendations for a standard serving. For example, the average pasta serving size is 480 percent larger—almost five times—than the USDA recommended serving size. This wouldn't be a big problem if people were taking home or pushing aside the extra, but several studies and surveys have indicated that most adults and children consume more food (and calories) when presented with bigger serving sizes.

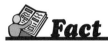 **Fact**

> In March 2004, McDonald's Corporation announced it was phasing out its "super-size" fries and drinks in a move towards providing customers with a menu supporting a "balanced lifestyle." First introduced in 1988, the seven-ounce serving of fries and thirty-two-ounce sodas have been criticized by nutritionists and health advocates for contributing to America's growing weight problems.

How do you keep portion creep from translating to weight gain for your child? One simple strategy is to encourage your child to split an entrée with another family member. Another is to order off the appetizer menu when appropriate and supplement that with a side salad or other side dish.

If you're lucky enough to have a favorite restaurant that offers half-size entrees at a lower price, take advantage. And if all else fails, order the regular, enormous portion for your child and ask the waitperson to wrap half of it before it even comes to the table. Filling the doggy bag first rather than last will lessen the possibility of your child eating past his appetite.

When to Pass on the Kids' Menu

But what about the kids' menu, you ask? Isn't that a more appropriately sized portion for your child? In some cases it may be—but the available choices aren't always the most nutritious. The traditional kids' menu items—macaroni and cheese, chicken nuggets, burger and fries, hot dog and fries, personal pizzas—can leave a lot to be desired.

If virtually everything on the kid's menu comes with a side of fries and a healthy dose of calories and fat, you can ask to substitute the fries with a side of veggies, applesauce, side salad, or a fruit cup. There's also no reason why your child has to be confined to the kids' menu if healthier fare is available among the adult offerings. Again, split a serving, or ask the waiter to wrap half for take-home before bringing it out.

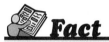

Fact

The Economic Research Service of the U.S. Department of Agriculture estimates that 91 billion pounds of food (or 26 percent of edible food available for U.S. consumption) ended up in the trash in 1995 due to consumer and foodservice waste. The ERS report cited increased portion sizes as one of the main causes.

Just Desserts

Another pitfall to the children's menu is that menu items often come bundled with desserts. This practice sets up the expectation that dessert is standard operating procedure. It can encourage your child to eat past his appetite just because the dessert is there. Even if dessert is a separate order, the choices are rarely stellar from a health perspective.

Dining out is often a special occasion for your child, so saying no to dessert—especially if others in your party are indulging—may not always be the best option. If you know the dessert will be a tempting one, tell your child she can have it if she orders light for the meal. Or ask for additional forks (or spoons) to split a particularly rich cake or ice cream treat among the other diners in your party. Again, the message is that desserts do have a time and place, as long as your child can adjust other aspects of her fitness plan—like the preceding meal or subsequent activity—accordingly.

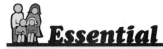 **Essential**

When your child screams for ice cream, you don't have to say no. There are many fat-free formulations of ice cream and frozen yogurt available, both in the stores and in popular ice cream chains. Many also provide a big boost of calcium. A one-cup serving (or two tennis-ball-sized scoops) is a good amount to satisfy your child and keep the calories under control.

Banish the Buffet

Buffets can be an invitation to disaster. Capitalizing on the idea that bigger is better, their expansive food offerings and bottomless plate policies give diners another reason to overeat. Even if reasonably healthy food choices are available at your local buffet, the unlimited quantities can spell trouble for your child.

Think about what it is about the buffet that appeals to your child, and try to find a suitable substitution elsewhere. Is it the opportunity to try new foods? Then be a little more adventuresome in your next dining experience, and try a new cuisine type. Does she like to have a little bit of everything? Visit a restaurant that serves a large variety of appetizers on small plates (also known as tapas, mezes, or cicchetti, depending on the cuisine) where she can do just that if you order several and share. If it's the supposed "value" that has you going back for more, remember that it isn't a deal if it's costing your family members their good health.

If you must dine at a buffet-style restaurant, start everyone at the salad bar first before moving on to potentially more dangerous territory like the pasta bar and make-your-own sundae station. Make it a family rule that everyone stays at the table until first servings are finished before going back for more, and then eat slowly. The extra time will give your child time to digest and decide if he's really still hungry or just entranced with the sight and smell of all that food.

CHAPTER 10

Learning to Get Physical

From the time they learn to crawl, kids are on the move. Inherently curious, and anxious to test the limits of their newfound mobility, most kids are running, climbing, and jumping as soon as they figure out how. Yet somewhere along the way, kids can lose interest in exercise. Maybe they decide it isn't important because they don't see Mom and Dad doing it. Or maybe their friends are more into television and video games than playing kickball and riding bikes. Reintroduce your child (and yourself) to the fun, and the good feelings, of fitness.

Fit for Life: Why Kids Need Exercise

Kids need exercise for the same reasons that adults do—to stay flexible, burn excess calories, build muscle, keep bones and joints healthy, boost the immune system, and strengthen the heart. Exercise also feels good, triggering the release of brain chemicals called endorphins that reduce stress, ease pain, and produce feelings of euphoria. Young children also need the challenge of exercise to develop their motor skills and hand/eye coordination. And exercise can be fun. Active kids' games, like hopscotch, jump rope, tag, and red light/green light, are important for social as well as physical growth, allowing kids to practice teamwork, sharing, and other relationship skills.

How Much?

Physical activity guidelines issued by the National Association for Sport and Physical Education (NASPE) recommend that elementary-school children get at least thirty to sixty minutes of age-appropriate and developmentally appropriate physical activity from a variety of activities on all, or most, days of the week. Better yet is up to several hours of cumulative physical activity daily. While activity can be spread throughout the day, the NASPE recommends that at least some of that activity be moderate to vigorous in intensity (aerobic exercise) and last for ten to fifteen or more consecutive minutes.

Aerobic exercise, the kind of heart-pumping exercise that increases both your circulation and respiration rate, burns fat. It is possible to overdo it. Your child is exercising at the right intensity if his heart rate is between 70 and 85 percent of maximum (see the section titled "Working Hard or Hardly Working?" on page 140 to find out how to calculate heart rate).

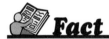 **Fact**

Anaerobic exercise builds muscle tissue rather than burning fat. Weight-lifting and certain floor exercises like pushups or abdominal crunches are considered anaerobic; they focus on exerting muscle groups rather than increasing heart rate. Because muscle tissue burns more calories than fat tissue, even at rest, low-intensity anaerobic exercise is also good for your child. (See Chapter 11 for special considerations and precautions regarding weight-lifting and children.)

Exercise and Childhood Development

Getting your child to exercise is more than a weight-loss tactic. Physical activity, and the mental stimulation and social interaction it provides, is important to the growth of the whole child in these four spheres of development:

- **Physical.** Of course, exercise burns calories and is integral to weight maintenance or loss. It also reduces the risk of Type 2 diabetes, raises HDL (or "good") cholesterol levels, and can lower blood pressure.
- **Mental.** Many sports engage the brains as well as the body. Players must develop a strategy to capitalize on their strengths and find their opponents' weak spots. Team members must figure out the most effective way to work together. There's a mental component to just about any activity you can think of. Even bowling requires some math skills.
- **Emotional.** Participation in exercise and fitness activities can impart a sense of achievement in your child and boost his self-esteem.
- **Social.** Team sports and fitness "games" require skills such as teamwork and cooperation, patience, empathy, and sharing.

Finding a Program That Works

The key to making fitness click is to find an activity your child enjoys. That may sound like a no-brainer, but it can take a lot of trial and error, time, expense, and frequent frustration to find that one sport or combination of activities your child can really get enthusiastic about. There are ways to whittle down the list so the task isn't so overwhelming. First, ask her what she might be interested in trying out. Then, think about her personality traits, and figure out what sports or activities might be a good match for the way her mind works.

Which of the following is your child:

- **Goal-oriented?** Something that offers measurable results, such as weight-training, cycling (with an odometer), or walking/running (with a pedometer) may be a good choice.
- **Impatient?** Long, drawn-out games like golf and baseball/softball are probably not going to be a hit. Try wrestling, swimming, inline skating, or even track events like shot put.
- **Self-conscious?** Individual instruction, or group instruction

with an individual focus, may be fitting (examples might be dance, martial arts, or fencing). She can also try at-home exercises like walking, jump rope, and mini-trampoline.

- **Competitive?** Then a team sport, or an individual sport that has an option for competitive meets, may be for her.

Don't invest a lot in equipment or uniforms until you're sure your child is enjoying the activity. Either rent or buy secondhand for those essentials such as safety helmets and pads that can't wait. You can find more information on safety and sports gear in Chapter 11.

 Essential

Sampling a variety of sports and activities can get expensive. Many martial arts academies and dance and gymnastics schools offer a free trial lesson. If a freebie isn't available, find out if you can pay for an individual class before committing your time and money to anything longer.

Make It Fun

Two keys to a lasting love of fitness in your child are variety and fun. Without them, your kids are bound to get bored. Fortunately, there are many easy ways to inject some entertainment value into family physical fitness. For example, try these activities for almost-guaranteed excitement:

- **Build some barriers.** Make your own backyard obstacle course.
- **Race.** Have a big family? Run some relay races. Or try those old picnic favorites, the sack race or the three-legged race.
- **Get wet.** Choose teams and lob water balloons. In the winter, have a snowball fight.

- **Hoop it up.** Challenge your child to a hula-hoop contest.
- **Go hunting.** Have a scavenger hunt with a list of unique outdoor items—fastest team wins.
- **Skip and jump.** Brush up on your old jump-rope rhymes, or draw a challenging hopscotch path to compete on.
- **Choose sides.** In team activities, pit the parents against the kids (with the appropriate handicapping to make it fair) or make it a girls versus boys event.

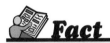
Fact

The park can provide an afternoon of active fun for younger children *and* their parents! Have a swinging contest, race on the monkey bars, or see how many times you can go down the slide in sixty seconds. Older kids can toss a Frisbee or a football.

Family Time

Depending on your child's age and personality, she will either find it incredibly entertaining or deathly embarrassing to have you trying out new fitness activities alongside her. Younger kids will probably enjoy one of the many parent/child fitness classes offered at local community centers and YMCAs. If classes aren't an option, try biking (or triking), swimming (or running through the sprinkler), or hiking (or walking around the neighborhood park).

If your preteen or teen is going through that embarrassment stage, you may ease her mortification by opting for active outings that are out of the public eye, like hiking and canoeing. She may also prefer to do some solitary workouts, and that's fine too.

Staying Safe

Before you start a previously inactive child on a new exercise routine, you should always get approval from your pediatrician or health-care provider. If she's starting a formal fitness program at a center or with a personal trainer, a doctor's note may be required before she can begin. Once you have her doctor's okay, make sure she has the appropriate safety equipment and clothing for her activity of choice.

Every workout should start with a warm-up session and stretches to minimize the chance of injury. A capable coach, instructor, or trainer should know the basics of warmups and cool-downs, but for parents and kids working out on their own, there are some rules you should follow.

Warming Up

Warming up before a workout is like starting your car five minutes before driving on a subzero winter day. It revs up the circulation of important fluids—oil in the case of the car, and blood in the case of the body—warms up the engine, and makes things more comfortable. When your child warms up, he actually is increasing his core body temperature and the temperature of his muscles, which makes them more flexible and increases his range of motion. A warmup also prepares him psychologically for the task ahead, which is particularly important if he is participating in a sport or activity requiring a certain degree of focus and mental alertness.

Some appropriate ways to get your child warmed up for a workout include simple calisthenics like jumping jacks, deep knee bends, and lunges; some quick sprints; a brisk walk; or a few minutes of jumping rope.

A good warmup will gradually increase your child's heart rate and her respiration (or breathing) rate, so that the bloodstream is carrying oxygen-rich blood to the muscles that need it. And while it shouldn't exhaust her, she should start to sweat. Perspiration is the body's natural cooling system, and a good warmup will get it started for the upcoming workout. Around five to ten minutes is usually a good average. If your child is working out in colder temperatures, the warmup should be a bit longer. Early morning warmups should also be slightly longer, as body temperature is lowest at this time of day.

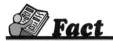

Fact

It is debatable whether stretching muscles before or after exercise will keep your child safe from injury. A study published in the March 2004 issue of *Medicine and Science in Sports and Exercise* found that there was insufficient evidence to conclude that stretching prevents injury in either competitive or recreational athletes. While further study on the subject is needed, proper stretching can't hurt. For some activities that demand flexibility, like gymnastics and yoga, it is essential.

Stretching

Stretching lengthens and loosens muscle fiber, and promotes flexibility. Stretching should always come *after* a warmup; stretching cold muscles can cause injury. Forget the "no-pain, no-gain" concept—stretches should not hurt. In fact, stretching to the point of discomfort can cause muscle damage. Hold each stretch for about thirty seconds. Again, a total of five to ten minutes of stretches should be adequate.

Here are a few simple stretches a child can do with you:

- **Neck and shoulder rolls.** Slowly roll your head in a circle, stretching the neck, first clockwise and then counterclockwise. For shoulder rolls, lift each shoulder up towards the ear, then rotate in a circular motion. This can be done forward and backward.
- **Lunge.** Step forward with the right foot, shifting your weight to that foot and keeping the left foot out straight behind you. You should feel the stretch in the back of the left leg. Hold for thirty seconds, then switch legs.
- **Toe touches.** Standing or sitting with legs straight, reach as far toward the toes as you can without pain and hold for thirty seconds.

- **Side stretches.** Standing with legs slightly apart, stretch your arms up in the air and reach for the sky. Hold for thirty seconds. With arms still up in the air, slowly lean toward the right, and then to the left as far as possible without pain. Hold for about thirty seconds on each side.
- **Lower back and hip stretch.** Lie on your back so that your lower back rests flat on the floor. Bend your knees, and pull them towards your chest. Hold for thirty seconds.

During stretches, you may notice your child try to hold his breath. Teach him that slow and steady breathing throughout the stretch is best. Stretches should be gradual and smooth to avoid muscle strain.

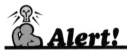

Alert!

Dehydration can put your child at risk for heat exhaustion and heat stroke. Research presented at the 2004 annual meeting of the American College of Sports Medicine found that two-thirds of children studied who participated in organized sports arrived at practice significantly dehydrated. Encourage your child to drink plenty of fluids before, during, and after exercise.

Personal Trainers

A personal trainer can be a great way to get your child's fitness program started off right. Look for someone who has experience working with kids, who is CPR and personal-trainer certified, and who carries liability insurance (either personal or through his or her employer). Someone with a communication style that clicks with your child is also essential. If at all possible, set up a short interview at the trainer's facility and bring your child along so you can get an idea of how the two of them connect.

A number of organizations provide accredited certification programs for personal trainers. These include the American College of Sports Medicine (ACSM), American Council on Exercise (ACE), National Strength and Conditioning Association (NSCA), National Academy of Sports Medicine (NASM), National Council on Strength and Fitness (NCSF), National Federation of Professional Trainers (NFPT), International Sports Sciences Association (ISSA), and Young Men's Christian Association (YMCA). Some of these organizations, such as the ISSA, provide training specialization programs in youth fitness as well. Any of these agencies can provide referrals to a trainer in your area. See Appendix B for contact information.

 Essential

According to the National Safe Kids Campaign, children between the ages of five and fourteen account for nearly 40 percent of all sports-related injuries treated in hospital emergency rooms. Overuse injury happens when tissue is repeatedly overstressed. It can be aggravated by improper or inadequate warmups before sports or exercise and is the cause of almost half of all sports injuries in middle- and high-school students.

Small Steps

If your child's idea of exercise is a walk from the bedroom to the family television, starting small is absolutely essential. You want to gradually ramp up his activity level by adding short daily doses of extra activity and keeping workouts low in intensity. A morning and evening walk of fifteen minutes each is a good beginning. Older children may be able to take on the responsibility of some more active chores, such as mowing the lawn, shoveling snow, washing the car, taking the dog for a long daily walk, or vacuuming. An appropriate increase in his allowance may be a good motivator.

Sometimes children are reluctant to get out and move due to embarrassment over their size or skill level or discomfort. Let your child know you understand how she's feeling, and don't force her into group or team situations. Instead, let her focus be your fitness program at home, where she has her family available as an emotional safety net.

Exercise should not hurt, so if joint or muscle pain is an issue, speak with your child's doctor. A low-impact exercise like swimming may be a better choice for your child. You may also want to get a referral to an exercise physiologist or sports medicine professional to put together a program that your child can be comfortable with.

Walk, Don't Ride

The single best way to add steps to your child's daily routine is to encourage him to walk whenever possible. The walk to and from school is a great start, but if that isn't feasible, there are plenty of other opportunities for you and your child to get walking. Next time you get in the car, think about whether you could walk to your destination instead. When you hit the mall together, park at the far end of the lot. Take the stairs instead of the elevator or escalator. Walk into a store, bank, or restaurant instead of using the drive-through. And choose family outings that involve more walking and less sitting, for instance, visit the zoo instead of seeing a movie. All these seemingly small steps add up—and you may find yourself saving a significant amount of gas, too.

Working Hard or Hardly Working?

How can your child tell if he's working out at a high enough level? Children between the ages of one and ten have an average resting heart rate of 60 to 140 beats per minute (bpm). Children over ten and most adults should have a resting heart rate of 60 to 100 bpm.

Again, if your child is breathing heavily but can still carry on a conversation, he is probably exercising at a moderate level of exertion. If he can sing, recite the Gettysburg Address, or argue with you while working out, he could turn up the effort a little bit. Higher-intensity exercise is probably best measured by assessing your child's heart rate during exercise.

First, determine your child's average maximum heart rate, which is calculated by subtracting his age from 220. Thus, a twelve-year-old has a maximum heart rate of 208. When exercising at a moderate level, your child wants to aim for a heart rate that is between 60 and 80 percent of the maximum. For the twelve-year-old, this would be between 125 and 166 bpm. High-intensity exercise should be 70 to 85 percent of the maximum heart rate, or 145 to 177 bpm in this example.

Although heart rate can be easily measured by teaching your child to find and time her pulse, a heart-rate monitor that straps to your child's wrist or arm may be a good investment and will provide him with a real-time view of his level of exertion.

 Essential

Teach your child to take her heart rate. Have her find her pulse at the wrist near the thumb by using both her index and middle fingers of the other hand. Once she's located the pulse, she should count the beats for thirty seconds (starting on a beat with the number 0). She can use her own wristwatch or time it with your assistance. Double that number, and she has her heart rate. The pulse can also be taken at the neck or chest.

Be Realistic

Your child will have his own individual preferences when it comes to sports and activities. While it's great to expose him to those that you enjoy, don't force the issue or express disappointment if they aren't his cup of tea. And don't limit his options by imposing your own gender biases. You may have a girl who adores ice hockey and a boy who loves to dance.

When your child does find an activity he likes, keep his involvement at the level he feels most comfortable with. He doesn't have to win every game or competition or move to the top ranks of the sport to reap the physical and emotional benefits of playing. If he's having fun, practicing good sportsmanship, and getting fit, he's already a champion. Encourage him without making him feel that he has to prove anything to anyone but himself.

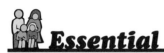

Essential

It's okay if your child occasionally wants to take a day off from bicycling or his other activity of choice. Just make sure his "rest day" doesn't render him completely immobile. Let him choose another family activity that is fun and active, like a trip to the beach or park.

Exercise and Activity Journals

The best way to both track your child's progress and keep her motivated is to have her keep an exercise journal where she can log her daily activities. This can be incorporated into her daily dietary journal or kept as a separate book. Initially, the book is used to gauge your child's baseline, or beginning fitness and activity levels. As she progresses, she can use it to challenge herself to higher levels of activity and physical achievements. It also serves as a constant reminder of the importance of daily exercise.

Filling in the Blanks

At a minimum, an activity journal should have entries for the date, type, and amount of activities performed throughout the day, and a total time tally for physical activity for the day. A space for personal notes may also be helpful; your child can use it to write down his thoughts on new activities he's sampling. Daily or weekly planners are ideal for this purpose, but a spiral notebook or loose-leaf paper in a binder or folder will work just as well. Leave a page for each day (more if your child is still learning to read and using pictures). It may make it easier on your child if you create labels for each section. For instance, you could have a section for exercise before school (what and how long); exercise at school (what and how long); exercise after school (what and how long). Older kids can also calculate how many calories they've burned each day, which also helps sharpen their math skills. **Table 10-1** offers some calculations of average calories burned during physical activities. See Appendix A for a sample activity journal entry.

Table 10-1: Average Calories Burned During Physical Activities	
Activity	**Calories Burned Per Hour**
Aerobic dancing	546
Basketball (recreational)	450
Bicycling (5 mph)	174
Bicycling (6 mph)	240
Bicycling (12 mph)	410
Bicycling (13 mph)	612
Canoeing (2.5 mph)	174
Circuit weight-training	756
Cross-country skiing (5 mph)	690
Football (touch)	498
Ice skating (9 mph)	384
Jogging (6 mph)	654
Jogging (5 ½ mph)	740
Jogging (7 mph)	920
Jumping rope	750
Gardening	323
Horseback riding (sitting to trot)	246

Average Calories Burned During Physical Activities (continued)	
Roller-skating (9 mph)	384
Running in place	650
Running (10 mph)	1280
Swimming (25 yds/min)	275
Swimming (50 yds/min)	500
Tennis (recreational singles)	450
Tennis (recreational doubles)	312
Volleyball (recreational)	264
Walking (2 mph)	198 to 240
Walking (3 mph)	320
Walking (4 ½ mph)	440

Source: National Institutes of Health. Based on calories burned for a 150-pound person. Calories burned will vary by body weight. More weight means more calories burned; less weight means fewer calories burned.

Reaching Goals

After your child has experienced a variety of different sports and workout routines and begins to focus on those activities he enjoys, he may find it helpful to add a "Goals" page to his journal. The idea is to make the new challenges both reachable and motivating. For example, a goal might be to ride his bike on a particularly hilly route without stopping, or to swim an extra length in the pool. As soon as the goal is achieved, he can establish a new one in his journal. This log of his personal bests provides a tangible record of the progress he's making, and it is a good source for reflection when he's feeling down or unmotivated.

The activity journal will only motivate your child if she remembers to write in it daily. Set aside a specific time each day to have her work on her activity journal, such as before bed or after dinner. The idea is to make it habitual so it's as natural as brushing her teeth before bed. A few months from now, when she looks back at where she was when she started this journey, and how far she's come, she'll be amazed at her progress.

Chapter 11

Integrating Exercise

Organized sports and activities, both school- and community-based, can provide your child with fitness opportunities that offer benefits beyond physical development, such as positive peer interaction and social skill-building. There are myriad fitness choices available, from team sports like soccer to individual pursuits such as skating. The key elements to your child's success include examining the choices together, gearing him up for safety, and supporting both your child and the programs he chooses.

Physical Education at School

School-based physical education is an important part of your child's fitness routine. The type of instruction she receives can instill either a lifelong love or an intense dislike of regular exercise. With any luck, she'll be guided by teachers who look at phys ed as an opportunity for nurturing each child's individual strengths, regardless of their skill level. Physical education should be fun. It should challenge without overwhelming and demonstrate why regular exercise is an important part of a healthy lifestyle.

Statistically, the amount of strenuous physical activity your child gets will drop dramatically as he reaches adolescence. The Surgeon General reports that nearly half of young people between the ages of twelve and twenty-one years of age are not vigorously active. Making fitness a focus at school during this time could help ensure that older children get the daily exercise they need. Yet national surveys show that schools loosen their requirements for participation in physical education significantly as children move past elementary school and into upper grade levels.

Is Phys Ed Making the Grade?

In the year 2000, the U.S. Centers for Disease Control released the results of their School Health Policies and Program Studies (SHPPS), a nationwide assessment of physical education, nutrition, and health education practices in U.S. schools. The SHPPS found that only 8 percent of elementary schools, 6.4 percent of middle or junior high schools, and 5.8 percent of senior high schools provide daily physical education or its equivalent—150 minutes per week for elementary schools, and 225 minutes per week for junior and senior high schools—throughout the school year for all grade levels.

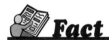 *Fact*

According to the SHPPS, 16.7 percent of elementary schools, 25.3 percent of middle or junior high schools, and 40 percent of senior high schools allow students to opt out of physical education courses completely if they meet specific requirements. This might include testing high on physical fitness exams, participating in community service, signing up for alternate approved coursework, taking vocational education, or participating in school sports.

According to the Surgeon General's Physical Activity and Health Report, less than one quarter (19 percent) of all high school students are physically active for twenty minutes or more, five days a week, in physical education classes. On average, daily enrollment in physical education classes dropped from 42 percent to 25 percent among high school students between 1991 and 1995.

As children grow older, the problem only gets worse. While about half of elementary schools require their students to take physical education, that number drops dramatically in middle and high school. By twelfth grade, phys ed participation has plummeted to a dismal 5.4 percent.

Percentage of Schools Requiring Physical Education (by Grade)			
Grade	Percentage	Grade	Percentage
K	39.7%	7	26.2%
1	50.6%	8	25.1%
2	50.5%	9	13.3%
3	51.3%	10	9.5%
4	51.5%	11	5.8%
5	50.4%	12	5.4%
6	32.2%		

Source: U.S. Centers for Disease Control

Standards and Abilities

How much physical education instruction your child receives, and the content and quality of that instruction, is determined at the state or district level. Your local board of education can provide details on the guidelines for your area.

The National Association for Sport and Physical Education has developed national standards for physical education instruction from kindergarten through twelfth grade. Some districts use these standards as a benchmark for their physical education programs, and many educators use them to guide class curriculum. The 2004 standards call for the following:

- At least sixty minutes, and up to several hours, of physical activity daily (at school and away).
- Limiting extended periods of inactivity (of two hours or more) during the day.

- Exposing youngsters to a wide variety of age-appropriate physical activities daily.
- Teaching children skills that are aimed at achieving lifelong healthy lifestyles and physical fitness.
- Encouraging self-monitoring of fitness so youngsters can see how active they are and set their own goals.
- Individualizing activity intensity based on each child's needs.
- Encouraging children to explore their unique physical talents.
- Nurturing character traits that foster good decision-making for children's health and well-being.

Making Positive Changes

Unfortunately, when money is tight in school districts, the first funding cuts are usually in physical education and the arts. Considering the already insufficient time spent on fitness in most schools and the growing problem of inactivity and excess weight in American children, further reductions in phys ed funding can be devastating to the student body in a very literal sense.

 Essential

You can also contribute your time and talents to your child's school. Volunteer to spearhead active student outings, such as developing a garden on school grounds, having a bike or skating safety event, or offering a fitness expo. Chapter 19 has more information on encouraging your child's school to provide adequate opportunities for physical fitness.

Parents can make a difference, however. Educate yourself on the physical education policies and funding realities in your school district. Let your child's school principal and other educators know that you support physical education in the schools, and attend your local school board meetings, as well as parent-teacher organization meetings. Encourage both educators and parents to investigate state and private grant opportunities that may fund physical education equipment or pilot programs. Finally, take your concerns to the political arena. Write your state and local representatives in support of increased physical education funding for your area schools. (See Appendix B for advocacy, legislative, and policy resources.)

Team Sports

Football, soccer, hockey, basketball, t-ball, baseball, rugby, wrestling, softball, volleyball—today's kids have many options to choose from. Team sports, either school-sanctioned or community-based, can be a wonderful opportunity for your child to get regular exercise and improve coordination and motor skills. With a good coach and a positive peer environment, team sports can also help build self-esteem and develop social and leadership skills.

However, team sports aren't for everyone. Your child may feel self-conscious about her size and skill level. If she does not feel comfortable with the prospect of joining a team, don't force it. There are plenty of other options for her to exercise her body and mind.

Pros and Cons

If your child is on the fence about participating in a team sport, here are some factors you may want to consider. On the positive side are the following:

- **Being a team player.** Being part of a team means learning how to get along and work towards a common goal, a life skill critical for all children.
- **Building leaders.** Your child may also find she has a natural gift for motivating her teammates.
- **Committing to fitness.** When your child joins a team, she makes a commitment to attend regular practices and games. This can be a good motivator for kids who need structure and scheduling to integrate fitness into their lifestyle.

- **Developing strengths and working past weaknesses.** Your child may discover she's a powerful batter but not so hot when it comes to fielding. Other teammates may have the opposite issue. Coaches provide balance by helping players complement each other's strengths. They also will help your child capitalize on her strengths and develop her weaker areas.

On the negative side are these factors:

- **Choosing sides.** If you've been on the receiving end of being picked last for a team sport, you know what a miserable feeling it can be. Letting kids choose teams is simply not a good practice for a phys ed teacher or coach.
- **Stiff competition.** Depending on the setting, the competitiveness in a team sport can quickly extinguish your child's excitement about participating. This is especially true if she is just learning the game and is less skilled than her teammates.
- **Warming the bench.** Ideally, all children will get their fair share of playing time. But depending on the setting, the coach, and your child's skill level, she could spend more time on the sidelines than in the game.

Teaming Up Outside the Schoolyard

When school-sanctioned team sports are either not available or not a good choice for your child, look into community-based options. Community centers, park districts, local churches, fitness centers (such as the YMCA), and area Boys and Girls Clubs are good places to start. Your child's physical education teacher is also a good source of information on what's available in your town.

Teams are usually structured around age or skill level or a combination of the two. This can be an issue if your older child is starting out in a sport and doesn't feel comfortable being stuck with the little kids. Conversely, your child may be placed on a team based on age, where his teammates are all playing at a higher skill level even though he is just becoming familiar with the game. Some individual coaching or instruction could be an answer to this dilemma. Talking to the potential coach about these issues is the best way to figure out how to address them.

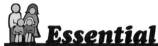
Essential

Remember that your child's overall experience with team sports will depend largely on the coaching staff. Don't hesitate to call up the coach and ask questions about her philosophy on working with kids. You can also make known any concerns about your child's well-being. A good coach will take the time to discuss her methods and address any apprehensions you may have.

Aerobic Training

Aerobics may bring to mind complicated floor routines taught by svelte, spandex-clad instructors. Aerobic training, however, is much more than this. It's the heart-pumping, vigorous exercise that burns fat, so a certain amount is important for your fitness program. Some good aerobic exercises include bicycling, jogging or brisk walking, rowing, cross-country skiing, stair- or step-climbing, skating, tennis, and dance.

Some overweight children may have joint problems that make high-impact aerobic training difficult or painful. If this is the case, look into water aerobics as a means of getting a vigorous low-impact workout. If your child likes to swim, doing laps is also an effective form of aerobic exercise.

Younger kids will probably be bored with traditional floor aerobics, treadmills, or stationary bicycles. Try entertaining activities like jump rope or skip-it balls, a ball that is tethered to one ankle and spun in a circle while the child skips over it with his other foot. Younger kids also enjoy playing tag on hopping balls (the inflatable kind that your child sits and bounces on).

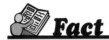 **Fact**

Because of the added resistance of their body mass, larger children burn off calories at a higher rate than children considered average weight who are doing the same activity. This is good news for kids trying to lose weight. The higher the intensity level of the exercise, the faster the calories are burned. However, if your child finds high-intensity exercise overwhelming or uncomfortable, it's better to lower the level and lengthen the time spent working out.

Strength and Flexibility

In addition to aerobic training, exercises that promote strength and flexibility can also make your child healthier and increase his sense of well-being. Resistance training builds muscle, and muscle tissue burns more calories than fat when active, making your child's workout even more effective. Flexibility exercises promote good posture, help loosen muscles and release stress, and may lower your child's risk of injury when he participates in more strenuous activities. Flexibility training can be as simple as basic stretches (discussed in Chapter 10), or a more formal method of instruction, such as tai chi or yoga.

Yoga for Kids

In addition to the flexibility benefits it offers, yoga is a great stress-buster for adolescents and can help kids develop mental focus. Even preschool and elementary school children find kid-geared yoga programs entertaining. The animal and nature asanas, or poses, allow them to become trees, lions, and other beasts. This appeals to their sense of creativity and imagination. Yoga is also great for developing their coordination and balance.

Because of its burgeoning popularity with adults, yoga classes are widely available. Look for a program or instructor that caters specifically to kids. If you have trouble finding yoga instruction for your child in your area, try contacting the Yoga Alliance at 877-964-2255 (*www.yogalliance.org*) or try YogaFinder online at *www.yogafinder.com*.

Start Slow with Strength Training

In their Policy Statement on Strength Training in Children and Adolescents, the American Academy of Pediatrics (AAP) recommends that children or adolescents interested in strength-training programs (those that build muscle through resistance training with weights, elastic tubing, or body weight) begin with no-weight, low-resistance exercises until they've mastered the proper technique: "When eight to fifteen repetitions can be performed, it is reasonable to add weight in small increments. Exercises should include all muscle groups and be performed through the full range of motion at each joint." Workouts should be at least twenty to thirty minutes long, two to four times per week.

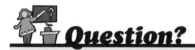

Question?

What is cross-training, and is it a good idea for my child?
Cross-training simply means mixing up the types of activity your child participates in. It is a particularly good idea if your child is easily bored. A cross-training program combines aerobic, strength, and flexibility exercises for a more varied and comprehensive workout—for instance, swimming one day, yoga another, and light weights the next. According to the American Academy of Orthopedic Surgeons, cross-training may prevent overuse injuries because it works a variety of muscles on an alternating basis.

The AAP also recommends that aerobic activity be added to a strength-training program for general health benefits. Heavy or "power" lifting and competitive weight lifting are not recommended for children and adolescents because of the risk of damage to growth plates on developing bones. As an alternative to free and machine weights, your child can try resistance exercises such as pushups, pull-ups, situps, deep knee bends, and abdominal crunches.

Solitary Sports

Kids who aren't into the team sport atmosphere also have a wide variety of activities to choose from. They can participate in activities they already know and enjoy, like biking or roller-blading, or they can take individual or group instruction in a brand new area. Yoga, martial arts, dance, swimming, kayaking, track, ice-skating, golf, and fencing are just a few activities that may appeal to your child.

While individual instruction may be more expensive than a group class, in some cases you may find it worth the investment to get your child off on the right foot and boost her self-confidence in her abilities. Later, when her comfort level is higher, she can join a group. Some solitary sports also offer your child the opportunity to participate in competitive meets and/or public performances if she's interested. If this isn't your child's cup of tea, find out if competing or performing is mandatory before enrolling her.

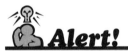

Alert!

Your child should never wear headphones or listen to a personal stereo when riding a bike or skating. It's also not a good idea if she's walking or jogging in a high-traffic area. Kids need to be able to hear approaching traffic, pedestrians, and other potential road (or sidewalk) hazards. The same rule applies for adults in the family.

Family Fitness

Make sure that your emphasis on fitness isn't a one-sided affair. Thinness is not a measure of physical fitness, and all of your children should be encouraged to lead an active lifestyle, not just the child with the weight problem. The same goes for all the adults in the household. Planning fun family activities that get everyone moving, such as hikes, trips to the park or beach, and family walks and bike rides, is the best way to demonstrate your commitment to your family's health.

For kids who prefer to spend most of their fitness time in either team sports or group instruction with their peers, your support is still important. Don't just drop off and pick up. Stay for practice, games, and competitions, and consider volunteering to help out wherever needed. Let your child see you taking an interest in your own fitness as well. Whether it be regular visits to the gym or neighborhood walks and bike rides, she needs you to set an example she can be inspired by and follow.

Gear Up

No matter what sport or activity your child chooses, make sure he has the proper equipment and clothing so he can participate in comfort and minimize the chance of any injuries. Secondhand equipment is fine and can save money—just be sure that it fits your child properly, is free of any cracks or tears, and that you check with the Consumer Safety Product Commission's (CSPC) running list of product recalls (on the Web at *www.cpsc.gov*) to ensure it hasn't been pulled from the market due to a defect or safety hazard. When in doubt as to the safety of any sports gear, err on the side of caution and buy new.

Safety Equipment—Head to Toe

Helmets are essential for any activity in which there is a potential for head injury, including football, cycling, skating, skateboarding, hockey, softball, and baseball. Make sure the helmet is the correct one for the sport, and see that it fits correctly according to the enclosed manufacturer's directions for use. Bicycle helmets should be safety-approved by the Consumer Products Safety Commission (CPSC); those that are will carry a label or sticker that indicates approval. Bicycle helmets can reduce the risk of head injury by up to 80 percent, so make sure your child always wears one, even if he's only taking a short ride.

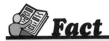 **Fact**

According to the National Safe Kids Campaign, traumatic brain injury is the leading cause of sports-related deaths. Of all traumatic brain injuries among U.S. children, 21 percent are sustained in sports and recreational activities, and nearly half of those are caused by bicycle, skating, and skateboard incidents. Kids who don't wear helmets or protective gear are more likely to sustain injuries than those who take proper precautions.

Other equipment your child may need includes the following items:

- **Goggles.** If your child wears glasses, he may require special protective goggles with shatterproof prescription lenses.
- **Mouth protection.** Certain sports, such as hockey and football, may require a mouth-guard to protect the teeth.
- **Padding.** Wrist-guards, knee and elbow pads, chest protectors, and face-masks are just a few of the available types of safety gear available for various sports. Your child may also need special equipment based on the position he plays on a team. Children who skate (board, inline, roller, or scooter) should always wear wrist, knee, and elbow protection as well as a properly fitting helmet.
- **Athletic cup.** Boys playing in a contact sport or an activity where injury to the groin is possible should wear an athletic cup both at practice and in competition.
- **Cleats and shoes.** Make sure your child wears appropriate footwear (including socks) for her activity of choice.

Secondhand shoes must fit properly to prevent potential injury and/or blisters.

Dress for Success

If a uniform is required, make sure it's a comfortable fit for your child. Take into account the extra bulk of protective padding when selecting a size. If you have to go into adult sizes, do so—if your child is uncomfortable, she won't be able to enjoy or participate fully in the sport. For activities in which your child gets to choose her own outfit, make sure she has a good selection of loose and comfortable clothing made of breathable fabrics that wick moisture away from the skin.

 Essential

While it's safest to keep kids out of heavy traffic areas after dark, older kids may want to ride their bikes, skate, or work out past dusk. Even in quiet residential areas, this can pose a risk. Make sure your older child wears light reflective clothing to stay safe. Reflective stickers on bicycle helmets, along with the proper reflectors and headlights on bicycles themselves, is also important to make sure motorists see your child clearly once the sun goes down.

Dress for the weather as well. For outdoor winter and fall activities, layered clothing works best. Your child can add or subtract layers to his comfort level. In warmer weather, dressing down is encouraged to prevent overheating. Just make sure your child has appropriate protection from the sun on exposed skin. The FDA recommends a broad-spectrum sunscreen with a sun protection factor (SPF) of at least 15. A hat can protect the scalp from sunburn as well.

Fitness for the Physically or Mentally Challenged Child

Under the federal Individuals with Disabilities Education Act (IDEA), the Americans with Disabilities Act (ADA), and Section 504 of the Rehabilitation Act of 1973, all children with a physical or mental disability have a right to full participation in a physical education program. This means that the school integrate your child into the general physical education program, or, if required, make a special adaptive program available for him. If a special program is necessary, the school district is responsible for covering all costs.

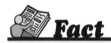 **Fact**

The IDEA defines a child with a disability as one "with mental retardation, hearing impairments (including deafness), speech or language impairments, visual impairments (including blindness), serious emotional disturbance, orthopedic impairments, autism, traumatic brain injury, other health impairments, or specific learning disabilities; and who, by reason thereof, needs special education and related services."

These laws also mandate that your child have access to any extracurricular activities the school offers. Specifically, activity providers must make "reasonable accommodations" for your child's participation. Although the definition of what constitutes "reasonable" may be a point of contention, generally it is any adjustment or provision of special equipment that does not impose an undue financial hardship on the school and does not endanger the health or safety of other students in the program. Has your school denied your child participation in extracurricular or fitness activities? An attorney with experience in disability law can help you determine whether the decision is in compliance with the ADA and other federal laws.

There are a number of national organizations and advocacy groups dedicated to the promotion of organized sports for the physically challenged. Turn to Appendix B for contact information for these programs and for information on disability law as it relates to your child's education.

CHAPTER 12

Emotional Eating

S ometimes kids eat for the wrong reasons—to occupy them when they're bored, to take their minds off troubles at home, or to forget hurt feelings. When food becomes a form of self-medication, it has the potential to be just as destructive as drugs or alcohol. Your overweight child also faces difficult emotional obstacles from the outside. Teasing from peers and even adults may make her depressed and/or stressed, and that can be a hindrance to her fitness efforts. As a parent, you need to be aware of the warning signs that her weight is affecting her emotional health so that she can develop the coping skills she needs to be mentally as well as physically fit.

Realistic Body Image

"Love yourself" is a message you really need to drive home to your children. A child who ties her self-worth to her body size won't be truly happy at any weight. But when popular culture propagates the message that fat is bad from an early age, it can be a hard attitude to combat. The problem is compounded by images of impossibly per-fect bodies that bombard children every time they turn on the television or pick up a magazine.

Expose your child to role models with healthy body types, in a wide variety of shapes and sizes, to instill a positive body image. Teaching your child to celebrate physical diversity will benefit her in other areas of her life as well.

For older children and adolescents, it's a good idea to start a dialogue about how the media, and advertising in particular, works to shape our opinions about body image. Children and adolescents are especially susceptible to the overriding themes in American culture that thin is in and fat is ugly (which they perceive as a judgment of their own self-worth). Teach your child to evaluate what he sees in magazines and on television with a critical eye and to understand how marketing and mass media shape popular conceptions of "beauty." Appendix B has some excellent resources for educating children about media literacy.

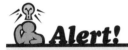

Alert!

The average fashion model weighs over 20 percent less than the recommended healthy body weight for height. In addition, the images of models seen on magazine covers and video are the result of hours of makeup and hairstyling, computer enhancement, and airbrushing. Let your child know the reality behind the image.

Fitness As a State of Mind

Emphasize to your child that weight is about having a healthy body and feeling strong, not about appearance. His size won't change his inherent value as a person and won't change the kid he is inside. As hard as it may be, try not to use the scale to keep score as your child works towards his fitness goals. By themselves, the numbers won't always tell the whole story. If your child is having a growth spurt, his weight loss or maintenance may be stalled temporarily. On some days, a bad night's sleep or a big test at school may make walking an extra mile extra difficult. You don't want your child to be unnecessarily discouraged if he can't always exceed his previous achievements.

It's also true that some children are motivated by the challenge of beating their personal best. Let your child take the lead if she wants to track her own progress, but stress that the numbers aren't as important as persistence and dedication to her health. And remind yourself that numbers on the scale and the pedometer aren't the ultimate measure of success. Instead, it's the pride she takes in her efforts and the improvements in her physical well-being and stamina.

Mindful Eating

As video, gaming, movie, television, and computer screens infiltrate more and more of your child's waking hours, the opportunities for eating (and overeating) without thinking increase. Eating in front of any visual distraction means your child's mind is not fully engaged in eating. He will take less pleasure in his food and may frequently eat more than he even wanted simply because he isn't paying attention. Meals should not be a multitasking event. Get your child in the habit of sitting down at the table and not the television so he can truly enjoy his food.

 Essential

For people with weight issues, the TV tray is among the worst inventions of the twentieth century, surpassed only by the deep-fryer and all-you-can-eat buffet. Eating in front of any kind of screen detracts from the enjoyment of the meal itself, encourages overeating by distracting you from your internal hunger and satiety cues, and prevents you from engaging in one of the biggest benefits of meal time, social interaction with your family.

Instruct your child in the first principle of mindful eating, which is to ask yourself if you're really hungry. Kids will often grab a snack because they're bored, upset, or even tired. Reinforce the idea that hunger is the only legitimate reason for eating.

Meals and snacks are also more enjoyable when they look appealing. Put the crackers in a bowl instead of throwing the box on the table. Unless it's a picnic, skip the paper and plastic tableware. Perhaps most important is to sit with your child (even if you aren't eating) and have a conversation. Make it a meal rather than a pit stop.

Eating Disorders and the Overweight

When parents hear the words "eating disorder," they typically think of anorexia or bulimia and excessive thinness. With these complex emotional disorders, food and weight become a source of power for someone who feels out of control. But eating disorders occur in the overweight, too, when food becomes a panacea to soothe anxiety and emotional distress. In these cases, your child needs professional counseling to uncover the root of the problem and learn healthier ways of dealing with it.

Binge-Eating Disorder

People with binge-eating disorder, or BED, eat excessive amounts of food in short periods of time (binges). Unlike bulimia, which is also characterized by binges, those with BED don't purge, or vomit, afterward. Thus, most people with BED are overweight or obese. Excessive stress or emotional upheaval are often triggers for binges.

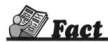 **Fact**

Binge-eating disorder affects up to 2 percent of adolescents, and the average age of onset is seventeen. The disorder is more prevalent in the overweight. The National Institutes of Mental Health report that among those mildly obese Americans enrolled in weight-loss programs, up to 15 percent report having BED, and the incidence is even higher for the morbidly obese.

A binge is characterized by uncontrolled eating, and a child with BED will eat past any hunger to the point of discomfort. During the binge, there is a feeling of complete powerlessness to stop eating. Usually the bingeing is secretive, and parents may be completely unaware of what is going on for some time.

BED is most common in adolescents and young adults. It also occurs more frequently among those with a history of compulsive behaviors and those suffering from depression, personality disorders, or post-traumatic stress disorder.

Recognize the Symptoms

A deep sense of shame and guilt over the bingeing behavior is part of BED, so if your child is bingeing, he will likely do his best to hide it. Some warning signs that your child may be bingeing include the following:

- Unexplained disappearance of entire packages of food from the refrigerator or pantry
- Hidden food in your child's room
- Weight gain when your child eats very little at meals, or other unusual weight fluctuations
- Evidence of frequent late-night trips to the kitchen
- A tendency to gobble down food quickly
- Signs of emotional distress, such as excessive sadness, irritability, or anger

Getting Help

Many people with BED binge as a coping mechanism, in order to deal with stress. Effective treatment depends on the ability to develop healthier coping strategies. Individual psychotherapy or counseling, cognitive-behavioral therapy, and group therapy are several common treatment methods.

Cognitive-behavioral therapy (or CBT) focuses on changing the thoughts and behaviors behind the bingeing rather than attempting to uncover the psychological roots of the problem. Distorted thinking patterns—"Bingeing will help me feel better" or "I'm worthless because I'm overweight"—are uncovered through exercises like journaling and role-playing, and the therapist and patient work together to build new and healthier thought patterns. CBT may be done individually or in a group setting. Group therapy can be helpful in providing additional social support for your child as she realizes she isn't alone.

If you suspect your child may have binge-eating disorder, talk to his pediatrician or health-care provider as soon as possible for a referral to a qualified mental health professional. When BED occurs in overweight children, getting a handle on their weight issue by normalizing their eating patterns is also an important part of treating the disorder. Your child's pediatrician and her mental health-care provider can work together with you and your child to develop an effective treatment program that addresses both the weight and the BED.

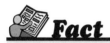 **Fact**

The prevalence of depression is high among people with binge-eating disorder. Children who no longer take an interest in activities they previously enjoyed and who become unusually sad or irritable may also be suffering from depression. See "Beating the Blues: Weight and Depression" on page 174, for more details.

Sticks and Stones

Words do hurt, and overweight children are a prime target for teasing. Kids with weight problems often feel socially isolated. They also tend to have a low sense of self-esteem, which makes taunts about their weight even more painful. Working within the school system and other social networks to improve tolerance and acceptance of diversity is one way to help curb hurtful peer behavior. So is increasing adult sensitivity to more subtle forms of negative and judgmental language.

While you can't always stop name calling, you can help your child deal with it better by boosting his self-confidence and teaching him how to react (or not react) to persistent teasing. You can also explore other outlets where he might find more positive social experiences, such as scouting, church youth groups, and volunteer opportunities.

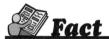 **Fact**

A 2003 study of the emotional impact of weight-related teasing, published in the *Archives of Pediatrics & Adolescent Medicine,* found that out of 4,746 teenagers in seventh to twelfth grades, 30 percent of teenage girls and almost 25 percent of teenage boys reported being teased by their peers. Teens who were teased about their weight had lower self-esteem, a higher incidence of depression, and were two to three times more likely to think about or attempt suicide.

Peers Who Tease

Your child may not automatically tell you if there's a problem at school. She may feel embarrassed or feel that "telling" on the peer who is harassing her will make the situation worse. If your child appears to be upset or just isn't herself, engage her in a conversation and ask if everything is all right. You may have to ask point blank, "Is someone picking on you?" To consider whether your child is showing signs that she may be the object of teasing at school, ask yourself these questions:

- Does your child seem withdrawn or sad?
- Is your child avoiding social situations?
- Does your child spend a lot of time at home by herself?
- Is your child staying home from school sick quite a bit, but is feeling fine on the weekends? (Do have your child checked by her pediatrician if this is the case.)

Your home should be a safe place for your child, one where cruel teasing and cutting comments are banned. But siblings are kids too, and they don't always see the consequences of their actions. Let your children know that there is zero tolerance in your household for name-calling, weight-related or otherwise.

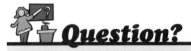 **Question?**

My son fakes stomachaches so he can get out of going to school. I think it's because he's getting teased about his weight. What should I do?

The stomachaches may actually be stress-related and the discomfort very real to your child. Talk to your son's teacher about what's been going on at school to see if you can determine what or who the problem is, and address it together. It's also a good idea to take him to the pediatrician to rule out any physical problems. Your son's doctor can also provide a referral to a counselor or child therapist who can help your child develop appropriate coping and stress-management skills.

When Adults Say Hurtful Things

"You'll never lose any weight if you keep stuffing your face the minute you get home from school."

"You definitely don't need that second helping."

"Another cookie? You won't be able to fit through the kitchen door soon!"

"Don't you want to be able to look nice for your graduation/ school picture/cousin's wedding?"

Teasing, both intentional and unintentional, doesn't come solely from kids. When adults say hurtful things, it's often in a misguided attempt to motivate a child toward changing his behavior. That strategy rarely works, and if it does, the emotional repercussions can be severe and lasting. Like any significant life change, weight loss is only successful if motivation is present from within. Most children are already highly motivated to get to a healthy weight when they understand that it will make them healthier and stronger. Far from motivating your child, the message sent is "You're a failure," "You're ugly," and "I'm disappointed in you." Your role, as a parent, is to support your child's efforts by giving her the tools she needs for a fit lifestyle and being a good role model. Ideally, the same goes for your child's teachers and other adults in her life too.

You will get frustrated occasionally. Watching your child suffer is the most difficult thing a parent faces. But when you feel upset and likely to something you shouldn't, take a step back. Ask yourself how you can say or do something constructive to help the situation. It's also a good opportunity to reassess your household for weight-loss stumbling blocks that could be hindering your child, such as a pantry full of cookies and chips. Again, you need to walk the walk, not just talk the talk.

Instead of saying, "You definitely don't need that second helping of pasta," try "Here's a little pasta. If you still feel hungry when you're finished, you can always have more." That serves as a reminder that your child should eat to her appetite only. Even better—ask if she'd like more broccoli with the pasta so if she's truly still hungry, she's getting her nutrients, too.

For parents of young children with weight issues, it can be easy to fall into the trap of labeling your child with "cute" names like "Chubby," "Little Piggy," or "Tummy Trouble." Don't do it, no matter how affectionately they are intended. Nicknames get ingrained surprisingly quickly, and they can shape the way your child perceives himself.

Helping Your Child Cope with Name Calling

It's a situation that all parents have to face at one point or another—their child is sobbing because someone made fun of him or said something mean and hurtful. It's heart-wrenching not to be able to just "kiss and make it better" as you once did. Your child's weight may unfortunately make him an easy target for insensitivity from his peers. While you can't fix things with a kiss, you can help your child develop some strategies for dealing with the problem.

It's incredibly tempting to teach your child the time-tested come-back, "Yes, but I can always lose weight. You'll be stupid all your life." But don't do it. Kids who tease others are trying to get a reaction, and further name-calling or insults will only escalate the situation. Instead, you might suggest that your child tell the teaser, "I don't like being called names," or "I don't appreciate it when people talk to me that way," and then walk away. That way she is taking a stand without letting her emotions take over. It may help to do a little role-playing and practice handling a teasing situation at home with your child. If your child feels uncomfortable responding, the best response is to just ignore the teasers. Eventually they'll get bored and move on to something else.

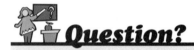 **Question?**

How should I deal with another child teasing my daughter about her weight?

If your daughter has made it clear to the other child that she doesn't like the name-calling, and she has also tried ignoring her with no suc-cess, it's time for you to step in and get involved. Talk to her teacher about the situation. She may have some insights for you, and you can work out a plan of action. If things don't improve after the teacher gets involved, it's time to take up the issue with the parents.

Emphasize to your child that the problem is not with her but with the person doing the name-calling. He should also know that it's okay (and not "tattling") to go and tell a grown-up if the teasing doesn't stop or escalates to the point where your child feels he is in danger. Bullying others is often a sign of deeper emotional problems going on with a child, so do alert a teacher or other school official if the problem is persistent.

While young children expect and need an adult to intervene in persistent teasing, an older child may suffer more harm than good by adult interference in a bullying situation. Adolescents are notoriously embarrassed by their parents—even parents who are just standing there breathing. In addition, the teasing may only get worse if the perpetrator finds out you've stepped in to try and stop the situation. A peer support group, or a professional counselor, may be better options if your child is mortified by the idea of you getting involved.

Finding Support

If the teasing problem is widespread, and it is causing your child significant emotional distress, talk to her guidance counselor, teacher, or principal about the possibility of sensitivity training in the schools. Your child's educators should be made aware of the connection between peer teasing and mental health issues, if they aren't already. See Chapter 19 for more on educating your schools about weight and fitness issues.

Check with your local hospitals, community centers, and healthcare providers about the availability of support groups geared specifically to overweight teens. Sometimes these may be in the context of a weight-loss program, such as Weight Watchers. See Chapter 7 for more on commercial weight-loss programs.

Stress Management

To most adults, stress is a grown-up affliction. Pressures at work, family demands, financial strains, and relationship issues can all cause emotional tensions that manifest themselves in psychological and physical problems. But being a kid is no walk in the park. Taking tests, a full extracurricular schedule, nightly homework, arguments with friends, and parental expectations can be a lot for a child to handle. When other concerns, such as a weight problem, are causing additional friction in a child's life, it's even more important that she has the emotional tools to help manage stress appropriately.

The Stress-Fat Connection

Stress does more than make you feel bad—it can also cause or worsen weight problems. The hypothalamus, the part of the brain that regulates appetite, is also part of a pathway known as the hypothalamic-pituitary-adrenal (or HPA) axis. When a stressful situation occurs, the hypothalamus sends signals to the pituitary gland, which secretes a hormone known as ACTH. The ACTH in turn triggers the secretion of the stress hormone cortisol by the adrenal glands.

Cortisol is called the stress hormone because it signals the liver to produce glucose, which generates the energy that would theoretically allow someone in a stressful situation to escape the source of danger. This survival mechanism works great when stress is temporary and short-lived. But when stress becomes chronic, the HPA axis goes into overdrive and produces too much cortisol. As a result, blood glucose and insulin levels become continuously high, resulting in increased fat accumulation around the abdomen. Other physical impairments, such as a lowered immune response, are also linked to chronic stress.

Is Your Child Stressed?

Many of the signs of childhood stress, such as an increase in time spent alone, irritability, and difficulty sleeping, are the same as those of childhood depression. In fact, the two may coexist. Physical manifestations of stress in children can include headaches, stomachaches, bed-wetting, and other sleep disturbances such as nightmares.

The younger your child, the more difficulty he may have articulating his feelings, which is why children under stress often respond by either withdrawing or acting out. Young children under stress may develop comfort habits like thumb-sucking, or they may become very clingy and upset at the prospect of separation from parents. Older children who are stressed often become emotionally volatile, displaying inappropriate anger or sadness. Stress may make kids of any age fidgety or unable to sit still and relax, as they dwell on the problems creating the tension.

Relieving the Pressure

Many times children experience stress because of what they perceive to be your lofty expectations of them. Sometimes those perceptions are accurate—parents do set unrealistic goals that can intimidate their children. It's an easy trap to fall into with weight and weight loss because it becomes a numbers game. Parents look at the weight charts and statistical graphs, pick the average for their child, and start the clock ticking to get them there. They fail to take each child's unique circumstances, physical build, activity level, and medical history into account.

Here are some ways to take the pressure off your child when it comes to weight management:

- **Stow the scale.** Don't subject your child to weekly weigh-ins. Let his sense of physical and mental well-being be the gauge of how well his fitness plan is working. If you must get out the scale, don't make it more than once a month.
- **Stop micromanaging.** Let your child make his own choices, as long as they don't compromise his safety. That means not ordering for him at restaurants and not debriefing him on food intake every time he returns home.
- **Don't overbook.** Extracurricular activities are great, but your child needs time for some unstructured rest and relaxation, too.
- **Emphasize effort.** Recognize his hard work, even if the end result isn't always what he, or you, had in mind.
- **Give them tools.** Practicing new skills like relaxation exercises, guided imagery, and yoga can help both children and adults relieve stress.
- **Lend an ear.** Ask your child how he's feeling when he seems upset, and really listen to his response. Never minimize his emotions, no matter how trivial the problem may seem to you.

One of the most important things you can do to lower your child's stress level and boost her sense of self-worth is to assure your child that you love her unconditionally, regardless of her size, grades, or athletic achievements.

Beating the Blues: Weight and Depression

Numerous studies have found an association between obesity and depression in both children and adults. Social exclusion and teasing caused by a child's weight problem certainly contribute to the problem, but research also points to a biological basis that both obesity and depression may share. Many depressed adults and children have elevated levels of the stress hormone cortisol, which can also contribute to weight gain.

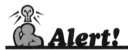

Alert!

A 2003 Duke University study found that children who were chronically overweight were at increased risk for depression and oppositional defiant disorder, a behavioral disorder characterized by hostility and disobedience towards adults and authority figures. Overweight boys in the study had a higher incidence of depression than overweight girls.

Weight and depression do have a symbiotic relationship. The fatigue, lack of interest in activity, and eating binges associated with depression can fuel weight gain, and further weight gain deepens the depression. Signs your child may be depressed include these:

- Sad and/or irritable mood
- Lack of interest or enjoyment in activities she once liked
- Trouble getting to sleep or sleeping too much
- Expressions of worthlessness or guilt, such as "I can't do anything right," or "It's my fault I'm so fat."

- Increased "alone" time or antisocial behavior
- Difficulty concentrating and remembering
- A change in appetite and/or weight
- Thoughts of or preoccupation with death, such as fantasizing about suicide or imaginative play with a persistent death theme

Often a slide in school performance as a result of these symptoms can be an early sign that your child is depressed. If your child is experiencing any of these symptoms persistently, take him to see his pediatrician immediately for a referral to a qualified pediatric mental health-care provider.

Getting Help

Once your child starts to reach a healthier body weight, it's quite possible her depressive symptoms could lift without other treatment. But because depression can hinder your child's fitness efforts, it's important to treat it early. There are several treatment options for depression in children and adolescents, ranging for psychosocial therapies to medication options.

In cognitive-behavioral therapy (or CBT), children are taught to recognize the faulty thought patterns that feed their depression and to alter their behavior to cope more effectively with them. Therapists use strategies such as social skills training, assertiveness training, relaxation exercises and guided imagery, and cognitive restructuring to develop a child's coping skills. Family therapy may also be recommended for working through some of the issues related to your child's depression. This kind of therapy may also be a useful forum for working out any family issues that could be hindering your child's weight loss problems, such as siblings who tease or grandparents who push inappropriate foods.

Antidepressant drugs known as selective serotonin reuptake inhibitors (or SSRIs) have also been studied as a treatment for childhood and adolescent depression. One SSRI, fluoxetine (Prozac), has been shown to reduce depressive symptoms with fewer adverse side effects than some of the other antidepressant drugs. However, insufficient research is available to determine the long-term safety of medications used for treating childhood depression. For that reason, antidepressants are usually a last-resort therapy for children not helped by nonpharmaceutical treatment.

Exercise and Mood Enhancement

Exercise is an effective, convenient, and clinically proven natural mood enhancer. Regular workouts can also improve your child's mood by giving her a sense of achievement and boosting her self-esteem. Unfortunately, when your child is depressed, it's likely that one of the last things she'll feel like doing is exercising. You can help with motivation several ways. For starters, take part in the activity. If you've made plans to do something together, she may be more likely to follow through with it. Make sure you choose something she has an interest in, and take baby steps—even a walk around the block is better than nothing at all. When you're first starting out, offer a reward other than food for the end of your workout. As time progresses, the mental and physical lift your child gets from exercising may be enough to motivate her.

 Essential

If your child avoids exercise with peers due to embarrassment, it's important to make up for that lost activity outside of school. There are a number of other fitness options that don't require an audience—hiking, biking, boating (as in rowing, kayaking, or canoeing), and weight training. Explore the options with your child, and get him started on a new adventure in fitness.

Many overweight children have a tendency to decrease their participation in physical education classes and athletics as a way of avoiding teasing and what they feel may be a humiliating situation. This leads to a self-perpetuating cycle of more inactivity and further weight problems.

Continue to involve the whole family in regular walks and other fitness activities as well as encouraging your child's solitary pursuits. Exercise is a great stress-buster as well as a mood-lifter.

Chapter 13

Through Thick and Thin: Building Healthy Relationships

As your child grows older, it becomes more and more important what his peers are doing, wearing, saying, and thinking of him. For better or for worse, this also plays a role in how he sees himself. Parents can play a part in fostering those healthy relationships that provide positive support instead of tearing down a child's self-image. When peer interactions develop that are volatile or hurtful, as they inevitably do at some point in every child's life, you can make sure your child is equipped with the coping skills and resources he needs to treat them appropriately.

Friendship in Childhood

A loving and supportive family is great, but parents and siblings can't be your child's entire social sphere. Forming healthy relationships with peers with whom your child can play, commiserate, talk, and just have fun is important to her emotional well-being and development. Yet kids with weight problems often face discrimination and bias at the hands of their peers. This is especially true as children move into the adolescent years where appearance issues and fitting in become of paramount importance.

It's great if your child already has a variety of positive and mutually rewarding friendships in her life. Do what you can to encourage these relationships. What about those that you don't approve of? Regardless of your feelings, give your child the autonomy to choose her own friends, and make those friends welcome in your home. Forbidding the relationship will be less effective than expressing your concerns to your child in a calm and nonjudgmental way.

If a "friend" starts to avoid your child after she's become the target of weight-related teasing, or says hurtful words, try to focus your child on more positive relationships in her life. With older children, you may be able to point out that this person probably wasn't a true friend to begin with. Talk to your child about what makes a good friendship. Tell her that true friends care about the person inside, and they demonstrate that caring through both their words and actions.

Popularity Contests

The teen years can be tough for even the best-adjusted kid. School is more demanding. Puberty brings a hormonal onslaught of physical and psychological changes, and what your peers think of you becomes close to the center of your existence.

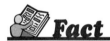 ***Fact***

The adolescent "fat stigma" found in the NLSAH also extended to those normal-weight teens who did count overweight peers as friends. These teens were considered less popular and had fewer friends than those adolescents who only listed normal-weight peers as friends.

For the better part of a century, American culture has hammered home the message that thin is desirable and attractive and fat is ugly. Being overweight is considered a weakness, a sign of a lack of self-control and discipline, or just plain gluttony. Yes, excess fat is unhealthy. So is cancer, but most adolescents would never think to ostracize a child with leukemia, while many don't give a second thought about calling an overweight child "fat" or excluding her from a party or get-together.

Just how bad is the problem? The National Longitudinal Study of Adolescent Health (NLSAH), a survey of over 90,000 kids aged thirteen to eighteen, found that adolescents who were overweight were more likely to be socially isolated than their normal-weight peers. When asked who their friends were, teens of average weight were less likely to mention overweight teens, even when those teens mentioned them. Overweight teens listed about the same number of friends as their average-weight peers, however, indicating that overweight teens were either overestimating their friendships or their normal-weight peers weren't acknowledging the friendships.

There's some good news to be found in all of this. The study also found that overweight kids were better adjusted socially, with more friends, when they were less socially reclusive and more involved in extracurricular or community activities than when they avoided contact with others. The message? Empower your child to believe in her abilities and to get involved with activities she likes for her own enjoyment, not to prove a point to anyone. Just by being herself, she can explode those myths about "fat kids" and show those peers who may hold preconceived notions about her just how wrong they are.

Developing a Peer Support Group

There are many options besides school for finding true and supportive friends. Church youth groups and community-based organizations are good starting places for your child to form positive new friendships. When those groups also promote volunteer work and community activism that she can take part in, they have the added benefit of giving your child a boost to her self-esteem.

A child who is having problems connecting socially with peers, or who just wants to find a friendly ear, may benefit from a support program for overweight kids or teens. Hospital- or clinic-based fitness and weight-control programs frequently offer some form of group therapy or support sessions as part of the program. A support group that focuses specifically on your child's age group may be useful in helping him develop new friendships with understanding peers.

When Your Child Is Picked On

Overweight kids are more likely to be bullied and teased than their average-weight peers, and kids who are bullied and teased are more likely to have disordered eating patterns and to suffer long-lasting emotional problems. Some studies have indicated that teasing actually reduces physical activity even further in already sedentary kids. Kids who are teased about their weight during sports and other activities report liking sports less and show greater levels of inactivity than those who aren't teased.

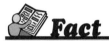 **Fact**

Bullying is more than just name-calling and physical intimidation. Subtler forms of bullying can be spreading rumors about another child or making negative comments that undermine his confidence—"You really are bad at softball, aren't you?" Other common forms of bullying include deliberately excluding a child from group activities and conversations. Make sure your child realizes this type of behavior is also unacceptable, and work with him to come up with an appropriate strategy for dealing with the situation.

A 2003 University of Minnesota study of 4,746 middle- and high-school adolescents found that those who were teased about their weight had low body satisfaction, low self-esteem, and high incidence of depressive symptoms. They also had more frequent suicide attempts and suicidal ideation (or thoughts of suicide). Teasing from more than one source was associated with more emotional problems than teasing that came from a single person. The same study found that among overweight children, 29 percent of girls and 18 percent of boys who experienced frequent teasing about their weight reported binge-eating behavior.

Clearly, teasing has a significantly negative impact on overweight kids and is yet another hurdle for them to overcome as they try to turn towards a more fit lifestyle. The classroom should be a safe, nurturing, and nonthreatening environment for all children. While you can take steps to help your child develop coping strategies, if problems at your child's school persist or seem to be widespread, talk with school officials about the possibility of instituting sensitivity training and/or bullying awareness workshops. Sensitivity training should focus on celebrating the diversity in all children—in terms of culture, religion, physical and mental abilities, and appearance—and not just be centered on weight issues, which could make your child feel even more stigmatized.

Letting Your Child Find His Way

Although it's painful to watch your child suffer as the result of hurtful words from peers, older kids need to learn how to handle teasing on their own terms. Acknowledge the validity of your child's feelings while letting her know that what really counts is the way she treats others and the person she shows herself to be through her thoughts, words, and actions—not her size or appearance. Engage in a discussion about what really motivates the person who is teasing her. Help her to understand that when kids tease others, it's usually because they feel insecure in their own self-worth and think that they can build themselves up by tearing others down. Make sure your child recognizes that losing weight won't gain them any friendships, or at least not any friendships that count. Of course, you should applaud any weight loss or fitness efforts she's currently engaged in, but don't imply that weight loss is the only way to stop taunting or ensure popularity.

Talk about positive ways to deal with the situation. If ignoring it is only escalating the situation, then standing up to the teaser (with strong but positive words) may be the answer. Do some role-playing, and try different strategies.

Perhaps you remember your own experiences with a bully or a persistent teaser as a child. Even if you weren't teased a lot, most parents have at least one story that they can relate to a child. Let your child know you've been there too and understand what he's going through. Tell him about a similar situation you were in, either as a child or an adult, and how you felt about and dealt with the situation. If your approach at the time wasn't very positive, talk about why it wasn't and how you could have handled it better.

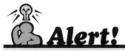

Alert!

Keep your eyes open for signs that the teasing may be taking an emotional toll on your child. Sudden bouts of stomachaches, requests to stay home from school, withdrawal, moodiness, and other uncharacteristic behaviors are a sign that you need to step in and talk to your child's teacher, guidance counselor, or principal.

Knowing When to Step In

Younger children have limited emotional and cognitive resources for dealing with bullies. If your young child is being teased or bullied at school, tell her to first tell the perpetrator to stop it and then to walk away. If it keeps up, she should always be encouraged to tell a grown-up about the problem. Children of all ages should be instructed to find an adult the moment they feel physically threatened in a bullying situation.

Be open and honest about your concerns with your child, and let her know you're there to help and not to embarrass her or set her up for further taunting. If your older child strongly objects to your involvement, then talk about what steps the two of you can take that are acceptable to her, such as getting her involved in a peer support group.

Fitness Camps and Programs

Summer means three months without school and a whole lot of opportunity for both positive changes and serious setbacks. Some parents see this time as the perfect chance for their child to really focus on health goals in a structured setting—a fitness or weight-loss camp.

Most fitness or weight loss camps are residential, or overnight, and do not take very young children. Usually seven or eight is the minimum age to participate in a residential camp, although policies vary by facility. There are also co-ed and gender-specific programs and camp programs that are divided by age range.

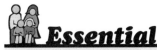

Essential

Be wary of summer camp programs that promise dramatic weight loss for your child. Losing too much weight in just a few weeks could be potentially dangerous for your child. A crash weight-loss program that focuses on the scale will not teach your child the essential lesson that fitness is about how she feels, and that eating well and getting regular exercise is a lifetime mission and not a summer task.

Is a residential fitness or weight loss camp a good fit for your child? If your child has attended camp before and enjoyed the experience, a quality fitness camp program may be just the thing he needs to get him on the road to good health. The answer may be less clear for younger children and for kids who either haven't been to camp or have been and didn't like it. Looking at the pros and cons, and talking with your child about potential programs, can help you decide.

Pros and Cons of Fitness Camp

The number-one goal of a good child fitness camp should be to provide a safe and supportive environment for positive lifestyle changes. That should include giving kids the tools they need to make those changes, including education about nutrition and portion sizes, instruction in physical fitness skills, and insight into psychological issues such as impulsive or mindless eating.

Beware of camps that mandate regular weigh-ins, highly restrictive menus, and before-and-after photos. These are all good signs that they're looking more at playing the numbers game than at making lasting changes for your child's health.

Even the best and most highly recommended camps have their positive and negative points. The pros include the following:

- **No cliques.** Most of the other campers your child will meet will also be new, so the social barriers that may exist at home or in other regular camp situations are gone.
- **Common goals.** All campers have a common goal and can empathize with what the others are going through.
- **No temptations.** Everyone shares nutritionally balanced, healthy meals without the specter of s'mores and Oreos lurking nearby.
- **Active fun.** Camp of any kind typically doesn't have televisions and video games, instead exposing kids to a variety of activities in the great outdoors. It's a great place for your child to sample a number of new sports in a nonthreatening environment.

The cons include the following:

- **Expense.** Fitness and weight-loss camps are not cheap.
- **Unrealistic expectations.** Camps that promise dramatic weight loss may disappoint and could even endanger your child's health.
- **Separation anxiety.** If your child attends a resident camp far from home, most of the friendships she develops with other kids who relate to her weight issues will have to end as the summer draws to a close.
- **A virtual reality.** Without the proper focus on skills training and how to eat and exercise right in the "real world," where temptation abounds, kids can easily relapse into old habits after leaving the sheltered environment of camp.

How to Choose a Camp

Camps should offer an open house or scheduled visitation for prospective campers and their parents. This will give you and your child the opportunity to meet the staff, explore the grounds, learn more about camp programs, and ask questions of the camp director and counselors.

If you are committed to sending your child to a fitness camp, and there are no nearby facilities that you can realistically visit in advance due to time or financial considerations, ask for a telephone conference with the director or someone knowledgeable on staff. The camp should also be able to send you marketing materials (including plenty of pictures of the grounds and descriptions of offered programs) in advance so you can do your homework and have your questions ready.

 Essential

Ask the camp you are considering for references. They should be able to provide you with names and phone numbers of parents who have sent their children to the facility in the past and who are willing to speak with parents of prospective campers about their experiences.

It's good to choose a camp that is certified by the American Camping Association (ACA). This means that the camp has met up to 300 health and safety standards established by the ACA in the areas of health and wellness, site and food service, transportation, human resources (staffing), operations, and camp programs. However, remember that ACA certification has nothing to do with the fitness components of the camp program, such as the menu the children follow or any exercise guidelines beyond specific requirements for safety in aquatics programs.

In addition to checking on ACA accreditation, it's also a smart move to check with the state and/or local board of health where the camp is located and inquire about their last inspection date and any outstanding violations.

Here are a few things to look for in a camp:

- **Low camper-to-counselor ratio.** ACA recommendations vary by age, from a one-to-six ratio for seven- and eight-year-old campers to a one-to-twelve ratio for fifteen- to nineteen-year-olds.
- **Parental involvement.** A worthwhile fitness and/or weight-loss camp program will include some degree of education for parents as well as the kids, whether it's in the form of special parent weekends, open house events, or group sessions.
- **Professional guidance.** Does the camp have a registered dietitian (RD) on staff? Are the staff members that head up the fitness programs certified in their field (such as an exercise physiologist, certified personal trainer, or fitness instructor)? Is there a medical director on staff? What about a licensed counselor?
- **High staff-retention rate**. If counselors return year after year, they are more likely to be dedicated and enthusiastic teachers for your child.
- **Committed counselors.** Are any of the counselors former campers? What character traits does the camp look for in recruiting counselors?
- **Clear policies and procedures.** The camp rules should be laid out in black and white so you and your child know what's expected. Procedures should also be in place for emergency situations, accidents, and illnesses. It's also good to ask about discipline policies.
- **Director experience and involvement.** A seasoned director/owner who is involved in the day-to-day operation of the camp is often better than a "chain" camp run by people without a vested interest in the camp's success. Ask the director what his overall philosophy is towards child fitness and the camp's role in promoting it.
- **A positive fitness philosophy.** Most importantly, you want your

child's camp to look at your child's health and well-being as a primary concern. The focus should not be on melting away the pounds quickly but on promoting a healthy fundamental approach toward food and activity.

After-Camp Maintenance

So what happens after your child returns from camp, fitter, perhaps slimmer, and enthusiastic about his life changes? How you handle this transition time will make a tremendous impact on his long-term success.

Many camps offer some form of a follow-up program, which may be a weekend retreat, periodic support meetings, support by phone or e-mail, or a regular newsletter. Take advantage of these if they're available. Make sure that your child returns to a home full of healthy food, and offer her ample opportunity for exercise. You can't expect her to stick to her fitness program unless the rest of the family is willing to join in and walk the walk with her.

 Essential

While you can't control the type of reinforcement your child gets outside the home when she returns from camp, you can make sure that your family and friends praise her more for her newfound interest in working out and eating right and less for the way she looks. Messages like "You've really gotten good at swimming" and "It's great that you've learned to cook such healthy treats" acknowledge the hard work she's done and boost her self-esteem.

Self-Esteem and Positive Self-Image

Overweight kids often have self-esteem issues, particularly if they're victims of taunting or bullying at school. It bears repeating, yet again, that working on weight is about ensuring your child's physical and psychological well-being, not about being pretty or popular. Integrating healthy lifestyle habits into your child's daily life should take priority over the numbers on the scale. Putting undue emphasis on losing weight sends the message that losing weight is the most important aspect of your child's life, and it ties your child's value to his physical size.

It's hard to fight years of cultural conditioning about fat and obesity. Even with the best and most supportive parental efforts, children can sometimes hang on to a negative self-image. When you don't seem to be making headway with your child, and he appears depressed, disheartened, or anxious about his fitness efforts or life in general, a qualified therapist or counselor can be invaluable.

When a Therapist Can Help

For children with self-esteem issues, cognitive-behavioral therapy (or CBT) may be helpful. A therapist will work with your child to expose those faulty or irrational thought patterns (referred to as automatic thoughts) that are at the root of her poor self-image. A process called validity testing is used to expose automatic thoughts by requiring the child to defend those thoughts with facts and logic.

For example, a therapist might ask a child who ties his self-worth to his weight to come up with a list of things he is good at, such as playing the piano or excelling in math. Then the therapist might ask him to list the thin peers he knows and what they seem to be good, and not so good, at. Odds are that in a few of the areas where your child excels, his peers can't compete, and vice versa. These facts show that he does indeed have value, that value is not size-dependent. All kids have different strengths and weaknesses, but that doesn't make yours any less valuable as a person.

CBT also works on changing behavior patterns so your child has better coping strategies at her disposal. If she previously ran for the refrigerator every time a peer teased her, the therapist might model some different ways your child could react instead, or the two might role-play through the situation. Other common tools in CBT include daily journaling and cognitive rehearsal, in which a child mentally rehearses how to handle teasing so his response is automatic when the situation arises.

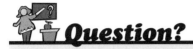

Question?

How can I find a good therapist for my child?
Child therapists may be psychiatrists, psychologists, or licensed social workers. Look for a licensed practitioner with specific training and education in treating children. Asking your child's pediatrician for a referral is a good first step. Prospective therapists should be willing to speak with you briefly either on the phone or at an office consultation to answer your questions and explain their treatment approach. This will also give you the opportunity to get a feel for how good of a fit an individual may be for your child's needs and personality.

Beyond cognitive-behavioral therapy, individual therapy may also focus on other aspects of skill-building or personal insight. A therapist might teach your child stress management and/or relaxation techniques to cope with anxiety. She might also use play with younger children to uncover the issues bothering your child and to allow your child to express herself in a more accessible way.

Family Therapy
Sometimes your child's individual therapist or counselor may suggest a few sessions of family therapy. This is a way of making sure everyone understands your child's needs and is committed to working together to support him. Family therapy can also be useful if there's discord or disagreement among family members and it's interfering with your child's weight loss efforts. Sometimes a neutral third party can be invaluable in providing a candid view of the family dynamics at work along with constructive suggestions on how to improve relationships among siblings or between parents and children.

To make family therapy most effective, everyone must commit to attending a minimum number of sessions and to trying the counselor's suggestions as the sessions progress, whatever those suggestions may be. Make sure this promise is made before the first session even begins—odds are that at least one family member is not going to agree with the counselor's take on things.

Someone to Look Up To

Many children don't live in a traditional two-parent household, and sometimes this can lead to a situation where they aren't getting enough support to either establish or work towards fitness and weight goals. In other situations, kids may have plenty of support at home, but they may still feel adrift when they're at school and have to make choices about what to do with their free time and how to handle social problems.

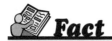 **Fact**

Over 200,000 American kids between the ages of five and eighteen participate in the Big Brothers Big Sisters program. Research has found that these children (called "Littles" in BBBS lingo) perform better in school and have more self-confidence. They come from all socioeconomic backgrounds and family structures. The only qualification for becoming a "Little" is that the child's guardian believes he or she could benefit from additional adult support. BBBS runs both in-school and community-based mentoring programs.

For the child who needs a little extra attention from an older child or adult, a mentoring program may be just the thing. Many are school-based, pairing up children with older kids or adults for regular sessions of one-on-one activities, games, and tutoring. These programs can form lifelong friendships, and they may also provide your child with an extra support outlet for her fitness goals. A child's sense of self-worth is often boosted by the idea that a "big kid" or adult wants to take time out of the day to be with him.

If the school district has a mentoring program available, and you think that a child in your life could benefit from the contact, see about getting him involved. When requesting a mentor for your child, you might suggest to the coordinator that he be matched up with someone who would enjoy and encourage more active play during together times, and who would be a good role model for a healthy and fit lifestyle.

Older Children As Mentors

Child-to-child mentor programs often work best when they are voluntary for the older children, so they are participating by choice rather than mandate. The program director or teachers in charge should also screen the children and explore the best matches for your child based on her needs and personality and those of the potential mentor.

Beyond providing a role model and a positive friendship, having a mentor who is "one of the big kids" at school may help your child cope better in the schoolyard. If any teasing is happening at school, an older buddy on the playground can often help defuse the situation simply with his or her presence. (If the situation deteriorates, however, or if the child is being persistently bullied, an adult should still be notified.)

Adult Mentors

For children of single-parent families or families in which a guardian, grandparent, or relative is raising a child, a friendship with an adult mentor can be a very rewarding experience. Mentors give kids another reliable and caring adult figure in their life to confide in and to turn to for guidance and support. Some mentors also tutor and work with children on academic issues. If an adult mentor program isn't available at school, contact the national Big Brothers and Big Sisters organization (online at *www.bbbsa.org* or by phone at 215-567-7000) about getting your child involved with a mentor in your area.

CHAPTER 14

Food and Fun

Parties, holidays, picnics, play dates—celebrations with friends and family are memories that your child will treasure into adulthood. Food is an expression of culture and tradition, and as such it figures prominently into these events. But when your child thinks of a family gathering or a friend's birthday party, is it the food or the fun that automatically comes to mind? Typically, it's the latter. Sometimes, though, adults have a way of making special occasions into an all-you-can-eat buffet. Celebrate friendship and traditions, and your child will be able to focus on what really matters—having a good time.

Making Fun the Focus

Special events for kids often center on treats and sweets. From birthday parties to family gatherings and holidays, it can be tough for children with weight issues to enjoy themselves. It's important to stress the friendship, family, and fun of those occasions and to provide healthy snack alternatives.

Remember that forbidding any particular food on a holiday spread is not the answer. Unless your child has food allergies, saying "no way" to something everyone around him is digging into will only frustrate him and make the forbidden food that much more attractive. A better approach is to limit portion size or allow your child to choose one selection from several rich desserts on the menu.

Above all, stress that parties are about enjoying time with friends, taking part in games and good conversation, and celebrating cultural heritage and family traditions. Food can of course be a part of that, but it should dominate neither the occasion nor your child's attention.

Handling Holidays

Getting through holidays requires a special blend of flexibility, creative thinking, and resolve. It's difficult to deny your child special treats on special days, especially those holidays in which food plays a prominent role. Rethinking the holiday menu to cut the fat while keeping the flavor will benefit everyone, so don't be afraid to experiment with old favorites.

Traditional dishes can often be cooked in healthier ways. For example, the egg- and cholesterol-heavy foods of Passover, like kugel and matzo balls, can be lightened up by using egg substitutes or egg whites only. The fat content in your Thanksgiving turkey can be trimmed down by roasting it on a rack and separating the fat from the juices before making the gravy (or skipping the gravy altogether, if you dare).

 Essential

Discourage grandparents and other relatives from giving candy to your child for holidays like Easter and Halloween. A soft stuffed bunny or a scary book make wonderful seasonal gifts and don't place extra temptations in front of your child.

The key to enjoying your holidays together is making sure the rules don't completely fly out the window for the day. Allowing or encouraging a binge will make it that much harder to get back on track once the celebration is over. Keep healthy eating and activity a priority, but allow your child to indulge in seasonal treats in moderation. And let your child know it's okay to say no to a host or another guest who is pushing seconds. It's important that he doesn't feel impolite or guilty for turning down food he isn't hungry for from well-intentioned but misguided relatives.

When You're the Host

Hosting a holiday gathering has its ups and downs. You can control your child's menu options and ensure she isn't overdoing it on inappropriate food, but you also have the often-tricky task of meeting the culinary expectations of your guests.

Sometimes the nature of the holiday and the guests will dictate or limit your menu options. If your great-great-grandma's fudge cake is a longstanding family tradition at Christmas, jettisoning it is probably not a wise choice. However, you can provide some additional healthier dessert options that your child can enjoy more of. Some more serving tips to help your child through the day include these:

- **Snack smart.** If you're serving appetizers or other predinner munchies, make sure you have some nutrient-dense choices such as raw veggies and low-fat dip to take the edge of your child's hunger once the more decadent meal items are available.
- **Keep it under wraps.** To avoid clandestine munching, don't leave plates of Christmas cookies and dishes of candy out everywhere. One platter of treats that can be refilled as necessary is all you need.
- **Serve centrally.** Keep everything in a central buffet location for the same reason.
- **Offer alternatives.** If old holiday standards are a must for your menu, make sure there's fruit salad to offset the fruitcake, and steamed veggies to counter the candied yams.
- **Clean up quick.** Remove the food as soon as the last diner is finished to prevent grazing.

Having the holiday at your place also gives you the opportunity to create some new and fit traditions of your own. Add an active element to your celebration that you think your child will enjoy. A Christmas caroling expedition can be a great way to get kids and adults off the couch and outside moving. Other holiday-themed activities to work off a big meal include Easter egg hunts and egg rolls, an evening walk to view holiday light displays, a Fourth of July parade through the neighborhood, a Thanksgiving game of flag football (or a jump in those fresh fall leaves), and a New Year's "resolution" walk to start off the year actively.

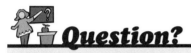

Question?

Am I being too harsh if I set limits on my four-year-old's dessert intake at Christmas?

All children—especially those in the preschool set—need boundaries to feel safe as they learn and grow. Letting your child go hog wild at the dessert table just because it's Christmas isn't giving him a gift, it's creating confusion and inconsistency in his knowledge of you and his world. Ignore in-laws who try to make you feel like a bad parent, and stick with the rules you've already established.

Keeping on Track Away from Home

For those holidays spent with family and friends, a few precautions will make the day both fun and fit for your child. Make sure he has a healthy and balanced breakfast the morning of the big day. Skipping a meal is the surest way to overeat all the wrong things once you get there. If the holiday meal is served buffet style, putting together a plate for your twelve-or-under child can ensure appropriate choices. Offer to bring along a low-fat, nutrient-rich food your child likes so you can be assured that there will be something on the menu he can enjoy freely.

Halloween: In a Class by Itself

As the sole holiday devoted to amassing large quantities of sugar-stuffed sweets, Halloween leads the pack of difficult holidays to help your overweight child through. Don't ban trick-or-treating or confiscate the loot bags. Do set up some guidelines for the holiday and its spoils, and give your child other outlets for enjoying the night.

Make the candy just one small component of the Halloween fun. If your community or local YMCA offers a Halloween party for children on the big night, spend a half-hour going door to door, and then pack the kids in the car and go enjoy the planned activities. Can't find any extra-spooky fun in your area? Set up your own haunted basement, or invite your child's friends over for a costume contest and bobbing for apples.

Setting Up Guidelines

Stem the tidal wave of incoming candy by limiting your child's trick-or-treating to only a few select neighbors or friends. It may be harder to keep tabs on older children who trick-or-treat without their parents. In this case, you can set a deadline for door-to-door knocking and then invite your child's friends back to your house after the curfew to continue the fun.

 Essential

Most children gather far more than they can (or should) possibly eat on Halloween. It's a reinforcement of the attitude that more is better, probably not the healthiest mindset for an overweight child. Limit trick-or-treating time, and if she's never tried it before, see if your child is interested in being the official door-answerer. She may enjoy passing out the candy more than gathering it since she'll be able to see all the costumes, make suitably spooky noises, and enjoy the feeling of giving rather than getting.

Of course, you should always examine your child's candy haul for any open wrappers or nonpackaged foods to ensure their safety. After you do that, it's a good time to go through and take out those treats that your child doesn't like or is indifferent towards to slim down their stash. Keep candy in the kitchen, not in the bedroom, to minimize temptation. Store it in a high cabinet or shelf where it is out of sight and mind, and where you can be the sole gatekeeper for doling out the treats.

Make this your standard operating procedure for all your children, not just those with weight issues. It's also a good idea to take this approach for other candy-intensive holidays, such as Valentine's Day and Easter.

 Essential

Want to get the bulk of the candy out of sight and out of mind for your child? Hold a Halloween Handoff, in which your child trades in treats for small toys, stickers, books, or other nonedible items. Take the Halloween candy out of the house to avoid further temptation. If you don't have any chocoholic coworkers to pass it off to, then throwing it away is your best course of action.

Offering Alternatives

Don't forget that Halloween is also about scary fun and great costumes. To limit trick-or-treating and candy overindulgence, host a Halloween party for your child. Top off a short trick-or-treating jaunt with pumpkin carving, ghost stories, costume contests, apple bobbing, and other spooky stuff. Let the kids and their friends build their own haunted house in the basement or garage. Or if you're really brave of heart, let your child and their friends stay up past the witching hour with a Halloween slumber party.

Smaller children may get overwhelmed by the scarier aspects of the holiday once the sun goes down, and they may be completely satisfied just visiting the next-door neighbors and calling it a night. Let them wear their costumes all day (and to school if it's allowed), and enjoy some at-home Halloween face-painting, crafts, and pumpkin-painting or carving. If they do enjoy trick-or-treating and still end up with more than they can or should handle, one way to make good use of the haul is to save a sizable portion for decorating your Christmas gingerbread houses a few months away. Since they're for show, not eating, freshness won't matter.

Movie Madness

The movie theater is a dangerous place for children and adults trying to watch their weight to make nutritious food choices. It's easy to overeat when engrossed in a movie; your mind is elsewhere as you're munching down the snacks. Large-sized popcorn comes in a tub that could feed a small army, with soda in a cup to match, and candy is in warehouse-club sized boxes.

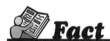 **Fact**

A large bucket of buttered popcorn (twenty cups) cooked in coconut oil contains a whopping 1,640 calories, 126 grams of total fat, and 73 grams of saturated fat. Sprinkle on a teaspoon of salt (which many chains have done already for you), and you'll have 2,400 mg of sodium as well. Add an extra-large (sixty-four–ounce) soda, and you're also adding 53 grams of sugar and bringing your caloric grand total to 2,440—just for one "snack."

In 1994, the Centers for Science in the Public Interest announced a highly publicized critique of the fat and sodium contents of movie-theater popcorn. CSPI canvassed twelve theaters in six national chains, purchasing popcorn samples and sending them to an independent lab for nutritional analysis. The results showed that most theaters in the survey were using either coconut oil (high in saturated fat) or partially hydrogenated canola shortening (containing trans fats) to pop their corn. Serving sizes were huge, and saturated fat content was astronomical.

Revisiting the issue almost ten years later, CSPI found that not a lot had changed in the movie concession industry. The majority of chains were still using coconut or partially hydrogenated canola oil to pop their popcorn. However, two regional chains they surveyed had switched to nonhydrogenated canola oil and sunflower oil, a healthy step forward for their movie-going patrons.

How do you find out what's in your child's popcorn bag? Asking the manager is a good first step, and it's something you can do over the phone in advance. You might also inquire about the butter topping (which is often more oil, rather than butter) and about sodium content, which is frequently high. If the news you get isn't good, bring air-popped in from home instead.

Strategies to Avoid Overeating

Never let your child go to the movies hungry. Grab a bite to eat before the show to satisfy his appetite so he won't be tempted to go hog wild at the snack bar. If you aren't sure of the offerings at the theater, bring some snacks from home. Individual boxes of raisins or other dried fruit, trail mix, and popcorn that has been air-popped or cooked in healthy vegetable or sunflower oil are some good finger foods to nibble on. You'll also save yourself a significant hit to the wallet if you pack your own treats.

If you do buy theater popcorn, skip the added fat and sodium of butter and salt, and split the bag or box so your child isn't tempted to double or triple her serving. The same goes for the industrial-sized candy.

Snack Bar Stamp of Approval

Some theaters have better snack options available if you know where to look. Larger theater complexes have started to add food courts with salads, sandwiches, soups, and other potentially healthier fare. Even if your local cineplex is snack-bar only, you can still find an item or two that will do in a pinch. Here are a few suggestions:

- **Baked soft pretzels.** Although the sodium content can be on the high side, this is one of the better snack bar choices. Just be sure to skip the liquid cheese (which is usually full of saturated fats).
- **Bottled water or juices.** Satisfy your thirst without all the sugar. If you choose the latter, go for a 100-percent juice choice.
- **Diet soda.** Artificially sweetened is a better selection than regular soda in terms of calories and sugar content.
- **Lighter sweet choices.** If your child has a sweet tooth, try trail mix or even chocolate-covered raisins to get some nutritional value out of the deal. Fat-free candy that takes time to eat, like licorice or gummy candies, may be more satisfying to your child. Just keep moderation in mind.

If you do buy at the snack bar, don't be "upsold" into extras. Concessionaires often combine popcorn, candy, and drinks into value packages. Unless you're feeding several people, these combos are rarely a deal—your child will end up eating more of what is of questionable nutritional value. Employees are trained to remind you that "for just fifty cents more" you can upgrade to the next size of popcorn. Remember—don't buy more than your child can or should eat. The health costs are too steep.

Fun Food Ideas

How do you make healthy food attractive to an uninterested or picky audience? To a certain extent, it's all in the presentation. Plunk a bowl of sliced strawberries and bananas down in front of a seven-year-old. Then offer her a strawberry-banana smoothie in a plastic coconut shell cup topped off with a paper umbrella. Guess which one she'll go for?

Party themes can sometimes make your job a little easier. If your child is enamored with horses, then trail mix, rolled-oat granola, apple-and-carrot salad, and horseshoe-shaped fruit bars are fun. Going with gymnastics or yoga? Try soft pretzel twists with a choice of toppings. Use your imagination, and adapt favorites to your party's needs.

Remember that you don't have to break the bank to pique your child's interest, nor do you have to be a professional party planner. Inject a little novelty into the menu, along with a healthy dose of kid involvement, and you'll have his interest in no time flat.

Tasty Party Treats

Kids enjoy creating their own culinary masterpieces, so make the party food interactive. Supply some imaginative and nutritious toppings, and have kids build their own personal pizzas on whole-wheat pita bread or English muffins. The same strategy can be used for soft tacos, another kid favorite. For the older crowd, make-your-own smoothies with a spread of favorite fruits and more exotic selections, such as kiwis and mangoes, can be a hit.

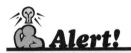

Alert!

For entrée fondues, substitute the traditional boiling oil (which can splatter and adds unnecessary fat to the meal) with a low-sodium broth and cook thinly sliced meat, poultry, seafood, and vegetable chunks. Typical dunking time is one to two minutes in the boiling broth, but always check meat and poultry for doneness before eating to avoid foodborne illness.

Fondue is another fun food kids can't resist. The name is exotic, they get to use their fingers, and it's the next best thing to cooking over the campfire. Entrée fondues, which are cooked at the table, can include just about any type of meat, poultry, seafood, or vegetable cut into chunks. Provide a wide array of dipping sauces to add zest to entrée fondues. Cheese fondue for dipping is also delicious; use low-fat cheeses for the fondue, and select whole-grain breads for dunking.

To go along with the birthday cake, let the kids crank up an old-fashioned ice-cream machine and create their own low-fat frozen yogurt or a light sorbet. Homemade snow cones are also a fun and cool treat. Use a variety of sugar-free syrups or 100-percent fruit juices for the flavoring.

Grab-and-Go Snacks

Blame it on the space program, but virtually everything you once ate with a spoon comes in tube or bar form these days. Tubes of yogurt, peanut butter, and applesauce can be healthful and filling treats, and certain cereal bars are also a good option. They also have the advantage of being packaged in single-serving sizes so your child can be conscious of how much he is eating. The downside is that the extra packaging typically means these products cost more, but generic versions are frequently available that can make the price difference less painful.

These are perfect snack choices to provide fun and utensil-free eating at beach party or picnic. For whatever reason, kids seem to prefer squirting food into their mouths rather than using the archaic spoon-to-mouth method. If your child has a take-it-or-leave-it attitude towards certain foods that could be part of a healthy diet, try changing the format to see if her interest is raised. Always check the nutrition facts label first—some of these products contain a lot of added sugars.

Food and Social Substitutions

If your child's social activities focus on food, it's time for a change of strategy. Video and pizza night is fine once or twice a month, but when it becomes a thrice-weekly event, you have a problem. Replace Friday night at the ice cream parlor with an evening of miniature golf or roller-skating. Rock climbing, ice-skating, swimming, skateboarding, biking—there are so many entertaining and active options for your child to explore.

Even if your child doesn't enjoy sports and prefers a good book to a basketball game, it's important to encourage options outside of television, movies, and video games. It's too easy to munch mindlessly when you're staring at a screen for entertainment, either with friends or alone. A trip to the go-cart track or an afternoon at the water slides, while not huge calorie burners, are an enjoyable way to engage your child in good fun with or without a friends and to get your family out in the fresh air and sunshine.

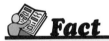**Fact**

Kids who aren't into athletics often find noncompetitive sports like karate and other martial arts a good outlet for making new friends and getting fit. Camping—and all the hiking, swimming, boating, and fishing it involves—is a fun way to get kids moving and interested in the outdoors.

Ice-Skating Instead of Ice Cream

Food as reward—just about every parent has done it at one time or another. Who hasn't made the promise of a cookie if your small child will just cooperate long enough to let you finish your grocery shopping, or a trip to a favorite ice cream spot after a stellar report card? Letting your child know you appreciate his hard work or are proud of his achievements is important, of course. But what he really wants is your love and attention, so why not make the reward that much better by enjoying a favorite activity with him? The next time your child impresses you, give her the choice of any one-on-one activity she'd like. Plan a picnic or at-home lunch together first to avoid food traps while you're out, then go hiking, skating, bowling, biking, or whatever else strikes her fancy.

Fitness Mixers

A great way to get your child active is to integrate fitness into his social life. Structured classes and team sports take one approach, but they may not be for everyone. Most kids love movement and outdoor play, but overweight children may feel shy or self-conscious about engaging in some fitness activities with peers. In addition, overly strenuous sports can be physically difficult and uncomfortable for anyone carrying around extra weight. Give your child ample opportunity to socialize in sports and activities in which his weight won't hold him back. Strength training, or lifting weights, is one good option. Your child should follow certain safety guidelines before engaging in this activity—see Chapter 11 for more information. Bowling is another activity that gets kids moving and isn't weight-sensitive. Golf (without the cart) will get your child outside and active.

Fostering Self-Control

You can't be at every party, school function, and social event your child attends. And even when you are nearby, your child needs to learn how to make his own dietary decisions. How do you ensure he makes the right ones (most of the time)?

For starters, make sure your child is well educated on healthy food selections. Children can and should visit a registered dietitian with you to learn more about what foods are the best-bet choices. Even the youngest children can learn about the food pyramid and what foods make their bodies healthy and strong.

Forbidding certain foods can make a birthday party or other special occasion uncomfortable and stressful for your child. He doesn't want to feel conspicuous among his peers, and the objective of the party is for him to enjoy himself, not agonize over what's going on his plate. So instead of saying "Skip the cake!" suggest small portion sizes that allow him a sampling of his favorites. Always encourage your child to eat to his appetite only. Before grabbing seconds, recommend that he take a ten- or fifteen-minute break to wait for his body to signal whether his stomach is full.

If your child is very young, you will probably be attending any parties with him and will be able to provide onsite guidance when the snacks and sweets come. But older children should always be given the autonomy to make their own choices. Chances are with all the distractions of party entertainment, friends, and other fun, they'll spend minimal time eating anyway.

CHAPTER 15

Sleep Essentials: Your Child's Body at Rest

From your child's viewpoint, there's too much to do and see in the world and too few waking hours to fit it all in. It's no wonder that she drags her feet when going to bed each night. But kids need adequate sleep to remain both physically and psychologically healthy, although how much and when will change as they mature. Chronic sleep deprivation can cause illness, accidental injury, behavioral problems, and difficulties learning and thinking clearly. It can also cause weight gain. So in a very literal sense, snoozing is key to losing.

Sleep Hygiene

Sleep hygiene is simply the maintenance of good sleep habits to ensure your child's health and well-being. How much sleep does your child need? The National Sleep Foundation recommends that between eighteen months and three years of age, kids get between twelve and fourteen hours each night. The required amount of sleep decreases with age. Three- to five-year-olds require between eleven and thirteen hours, and five- to twelve-year-olds need nine to eleven hours. Once your child hits the teen years, he needs an average of nine and a quarter hours of sleep each night.

To ensure your child gets the rest she needs, make sure her sleep environment is designed for a restful night's sleep. A quiet, comfortable, and cool bedroom is important. So are regularly established and consistent times for going to sleep and waking up.

Essential

Babies, toddlers, and preschoolers need their naps to get adequate sleep. Most children make the switch from two naps to one long nap at around eighteen months. At age three, 92 percent of toddlers are still enjoying a daily nap. That number drops to 57 percent by age four and 27 percent by age five.

Ensuring Good Sleep Habits

No matter what your child's age, there are some basic tenets you can follow to try and ensure she gets a good night's sleep. From the time she first sleeps through the night, you should work towards establishing a regular time for bed and a standard bedtime routine. Of course the routine will evolve over time, as your sixteen-year-old will probably not appreciate a bedtime story, but the basic purpose—of winding down your child and easing her out of the activities of the day and into the relaxation of sleep—remains the same.

Start the wind-down time about thirty minutes to an hour before bedtime. All television watching, video games, and physically vigorous play should stop, and your child should redirect her focus to things like reading or quiet play. If she requests a snack, make sure it doesn't contain any caffeine, and keep it light. Dairy foods are often good choices because they contain the natural sleep-enhancing amino acid tryptophan. A bath is sometimes a good way to relax your younger children for bedtime. Brushing teeth, washing up, and using the bathroom can be part of the ritual that signals your child that sleep-time is approaching.

Finally, try to keep your child's wake-up time as consistent as her bedtime. Sleeping in until noon on the weekend can throw off her internal clock and make it difficult to get back on track during the week. However, if she loses some sleep time during the week due to a big event, do let her catch an extra few hours' shut-eye when she can.

Circadian Rhythms

Circadian rhythms—also known variously as an internal clock, biological timer, or diurnal cycle—govern your child's sleep cycle. They are physiological patterns of sleep and wakefulness loosely based on a twenty-four–hour cycle and regulated by cues of light and darkness. When your child goes to bed late repeatedly or has difficulty falling asleep for whatever reason, he can unintentionally reset his circadian rhythm and have a hard time returning to an appropriate sleep schedule.

If your child is having problems getting to sleep, or she is suffering from excessive sleepiness during the day that isn't apnea related (described in the section titled "Sleep Apnea and Childhood Obesity," on page 213), her circadian rhythms may be off cycle and in need of resetting. Don't try to fix the problem by sending her to bed early. Regulating the time your child wakes up in the morning is the most important factor in correcting a circadian rhythm disorder. Wake her at a fixed time, even if she fell asleep late the night before, and expose her to bright lights for about forty-five minutes after waking (either sunlight or artificial light) to signal her body to reset the clock.

Children, Weight, and Sleep Problems

Your child's weight problem can influence his ability to get a good night's sleep. There's also some clinical evidence that a lack of proper sleep can contribute to weight gain, which could place your child in an endless sleepless-night/weight-gain cycle. And sleep deprivation has been linked to increased insulin resistance, a risk factor for and symptom of Type 2 diabetes.

A tired child is naturally less interested in and energized for exercise. Fatigue can affect cognitive function and impair your child's ability to make clear-headed decisions about food and other fitness-related choices. Overweight children are also at risk for obstructive sleep apnea, a condition that disrupts their breathing during the night and results in fitful or broken sleep.

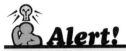

Alert!

While exercise in the morning or afternoon is thought to promote better sleep, exercise too close to bedtime can interfere with your child's ability to get to sleep. Refrain from vigorous aerobic activity up to four hours before bed. Exercise that promotes relaxation, such as some forms of yoga, is fine closer to bedtime.

Stages of Sleep

There are five stages of sleep that are differentiated by depth of sleep and brain wave patterns. The first stage is that initial five to ten minutes of drowsiness, or drifting off to sleep. Stage two is when the heart rate and brain waves slow and you are in light sleep. Stages three and four are considered deep sleep and are characterized by delta waves (also called slow-wave sleep). Finally, stage-five sleep is when dreaming occurs. This is also called REM, or rapid eye movement, sleep.

The stages cycle several times throughout a single sleep session. Sleep stages one through four usually last between ninety minutes to two hours, with each stage lasting anywhere from five to fifteen minutes. When the first REM sleep occurs, it only lasts a short time (about ten minutes). Then the cycle repeats, and the REM sleep periods grow progressively longer until they reach about an hour shortly before waking.

Children whose sleep cycles are cut short, or who repeatedly wake up during the night and don't get adequate deep sleep or REM sleep, can have problems with learning, concentration, mood swings, and memory. Long-term sleep deprivation also puts them at greater risk for heart disease.

More Homework

If your child seems to be having problems getting adequate sleep, it's a good idea to keep track of her sleep habits with a sleep diary over a period of a week. You can have her add the information to her fitness journal, which will also allow you to see how her sleep patterns influence her eating and exercise and vice versa. Include information on bedtime and wake-up times, how your child feels upon awakening (tired and irritable or rested and refreshed?), the number of times she recalls awakening in the night, if any, and her general mood and disposition during the day. Running a tape recorder in her room or using a baby monitor can help you detect possible snoring, which could be a sign of sleep apnea.

Sleep Apnea and Childhood Obesity

Obstructive sleep apnea is a disorder that results in a periodic inability to breathe during sleep due to an obstructed airway. Airways are often blocked by enlarged adenoids and/or tonsils. It is also happens frequently in overweight adults, with excess fat blocking the airway when the muscles supporting it relax during sleep. Unfortunately, overweight kids can get sleep apnea too. It can be even more debilitating in children than it is in adults because younger people require more sleep to function properly.

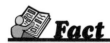 **Fact**

Obstructive hyponea occurs when the airway isn't completely blocked but is narrowed significantly, resulting in a 30- to 50-percent airflow reduction that also wakes the sleeper. Like obstructive apnea, it can be caused by weight problems and should be appropriately treated to restore proper sleep hygiene.

The hallmark feature of obstructive sleep apnea is periodic lapses in breathing as the airway becomes blocked. These pauses occur throughout the night, and the sleeper wakes up each time until breathing resumes. The result is a poor night's sleep and all the physical, emotional, and cognitive problems that come with chronic sleep deprivation.

Symptoms of sleep apnea may include the following:

- Nighttime snoring and mouth breathing
- Nighttime breathing pauses
- Nighttime restless sleep
- Nighttime sweating and/or bedwetting
- Nightmares or night terrors
- Difficulty waking up in the morning
- Daytime sleepiness
- Difficulty concentrating during the day
- Daytime hyperactivity and behavior problems

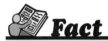 **Fact**

There are actually three types of sleep apnea—obstructive, central, and mixed. Only obstructive can be caused by weight problems. Central apnea is a rare neurological problem caused by a dysfunction in the central nervous system that stops breathing. Mixed apnea is a combination of both central and obstructive.

A sleep study (called polysomnography) conducted in a sleep clinic or with home monitoring equipment can determine if your child is suffering from obstructive sleep apnea. In some cases, surgery to remove tonsils and/or adenoids is suggested. A machine called a C-PAP (continuous positive airway pressure) may also be prescribed for your child to keep his airway open while he sleeps. If your doctor thinks the apnea is weight-related, getting your child on a fitness program and bringing his weight to a healthy level can resolve symptoms.

Stress, Anxiety, and Sleep Disorders

Does your child have racing thoughts she just can't still as she lies awake in bed? Cortisol, the stress hormone that accompanies chronic stress, can promote sleeplessness. If your child is anxious or upset about weight-related problems or other aspects of her life, the resulting stress can be causing her sleepless nights. Chronic stress and the elevated cortisol levels that come with it also increase appetite and have been linked to weight gain. Whether it be teasing at school or anxiety about an upcoming test, determining the cause of the stress is important in resolving your child's sleep difficulties. If it's something beyond her control, you might try some of the stress management solutions detailed in Chapter 12.

The Toll of Sleep Deprivation

The National Sleep Foundation estimates that sleep deprivation costs American business an estimated $18 billion annually in lost productivity. Drowsy driving accidents cost an additional $12.5 billion each year in lost productivity and property damage. For kids, the cost can also be dear—missed learning opportunities, diminished school performance, and sleep-related disease and illness.

Cognitive Impairments

Every parent knows that fuzzy-headed feeling that comes with an inadequate night's sleep. Whether you're at the staying-up-all-night-with-a-fussy-baby-stage, or in the waiting-up-for-a-teen-who's-out-past-curfew era, you know that a poor night's rest puts you off your game for the whole day. Your child may have even more at stake. His brain is developing, and he faces new tasks and opportunities to learn daily at school. If he's unable to concentrate and think clearly due to fatigue, he's going to miss out on those opportunities.

Clinical studies have linked sleep deprivation to poor performance on some memory tasks, contextual and abstract learning difficulties, delayed mental and physical reaction times, and changes in behavior and mood such as irritability, hyperactivity, and frustration. High school students who get lower grades also tend to get less sleep and have more irregular sleep patterns than their higher-achieving peers.

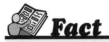 **Fact**

Over a quarter of adolescent students surveyed by the National Sleep Foundation reported that they get 6.5 hours of sleep or less per night—far less than the recommended 9.25 hours. Compounding this problem is the fact that once puberty arrives, teens have a naturally occurring shift in the timing of the melatonin release that signals the start of their sleep cycle. Their bedtimes naturally shift to later, yet they still have to get up at the same time for school, and they still require the same amount of sleep to function properly.

Physical Toll

Chronic sleep deprivation can also affect your child's body as well as her mind. It promotes insulin resistance (associated with Type 2 diabetes) and can weaken her immune system, making her more susceptible to infections. It can also impact hormone levels. Secretion of the hormone leptin, which helps regulate body fat and food intake, is synchronized by circadian rhythms. Lack of sleep lowers circulating leptin levels, and low leptin levels have been associated with weight gain and Type 2 diabetes.

Driving While Drowsy

The National Highway Traffic Safety Administration (NHTSA) attributes at least 100,000 traffic accidents annually to a driver who got behind the wheel without sufficient sleep. Teens and young adults between the ages of sixteen and twenty-nine, particularly males, are at highest risk being involved in a drowsy driving accident. Undiagnosed sleep apnea also increases risk. Parents should be just as vigilant about educating their driving teens about the dangers of falling asleep at the wheel as they are about talking about drinking and driving.

The delayed reaction times caused by sleep deprivation can be just as dangerous, if not more so, than driving under the influence of alcohol. A 2001 Queen's University study found that subjects kept awake for 18.5 and 21 hours had driving deficits similar to those subjects who had slept normally but imbibed to a blood alcohol concentration of .05 and .08 percent, respectively.

Eat Right, Sleep Tight

What your child snacks on before bed can keep her awake or help send her off to dreamland. Eating a particularly large, rich, or spicy meal too close to bedtime can make sleep difficult for your child. In fact, eating within an hour of bed can disrupt sleep, so ask your child about ninety minutes prior to curfew if she's going to want a bedtime snack.

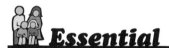

Essential

Combining both carbohydrates and calcium with tryptophan foods increases their availability in the bloodstream for transport into the brain. Avoid a high-protein/low-carb snack at bedtime as it will increase brain function rather than slow it down. Some good bedtime snack ideas for promoting sleep include a half a peanut butter sandwich on whole-grain bread with a glass of milk, hot or cold whole-grain cereal with milk, or a deviled egg with a side of milk.

Studies have indicated that the amino acid L-tryptophan, found in milk, turkey, beans, eggs, peanuts, seeds, and other foods, promotes sleep by enhancing the production of the neurotransmitter serotonin.

Another similar serotonin precursor, the amino acid L-5-hydroxytryp-tophan, was effective in resolving the sleep difficulties of children with night terrors in a University of Rome study.

Supplementing Sleep

Clinical studies have associated certain vitamin deficiencies with sleep problems. They have also pinpointed specific vitamin and mineral supplementation that has been found to help promote sleep. Here are some common vitamins and minerals that can influence the body's ability to sleep:

- **Vitamin B$_1$ (thiamine).** In studies of thiamine-deficient adults, supplementation with B1 reduced fatigue and improved sleep patterns.
- **Vitamin B$_{12}$.** Found in meat, fish, eggs, dairy products, and fortified cereals, B$_{12}$ has a regulating effect on circadian rhythms and may be helpful in adjusting your child's sleep cycle.
- **Magnesium.** Magnesium deficiency has been associated with several sleep disorders. Supplementation can promote sleep. Foods high in magnesium include spinach and other dark green veggies, tree nuts, soy, whole grains, and seeds.

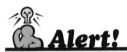

Alert!

If your child is having sleep problems, look at his caffeine intake from food and beverages (such as soda, tea, and chocolate drinks). The National Sleep Foundation recommends that both children and adults have no more than 250 mg of caffeine daily to avoid sleep problems. Try to avoid any caffeine intake beyond dinner so it isn't too close to bedtime, as well.

Melatonin is neither a vitamin nor a mineral. It is a hormone, available over the counter in supplement form, which can promote sleep. Melatonin is secreted by the pineal gland and helps to regulate your child's sleep cycles. Although pediatric studies on the supplement are still sparse, the supplement appears to be useful in children with few, if any, side effects.

Don't give your child vitamin supplements without first consulting his pediatrician. If his doctor suspects a vitamin deficiency, a simple blood test can usually confirm or rule out the diagnosis.

Improving the Sleep Environment

Your child's bedroom is his personal sanctuary, the place where he plays with his toys, entertains his friends, reads his books, writes down his private thoughts and dreams, and, of course, sleeps. Sometime it's a challenge to transform this multipurpose room into a restful and relaxing environment for sleep once the sun goes down.

Start with the basics—good bedding, appropriate lighting, and a quiet atmosphere. Then control those environmental elements that might cause unwanted stimulation too close to bedtime. Younger kids don't need televisions, DVD players, and video games in their rooms, as they present a distraction at bedtime. It may be unrealistic to ban a computer from an older child's room if he uses it for school, but you can put some limits on its use. You can also insist that all electronic items be powered down an hour or two before bedtime, at least. A radio or CD player is okay if it's used to play mellow music or white noise.

Bedroom Basics

Start off with a comfortable bed and mattress. If you still have your child in a toddler bed that he's really too big for, now's the time to invest in a big-kid bed. If your child is sleeping on a mattress that's been passed down from three older siblings, you might be wise to replace it. Look for a mattress and box spring set that's firm yet supportive. Take your child shopping with you, and let him test-drive the choices in the store. And let him pick out a set of soft sheets in colors he likes to make bedtime more appealing.

It's more difficult to sleep in a room that's too warm, so ensure that your child has adequate ventilation in the summer months. A good rule-of-thumb temperature zone for comfortable sleep is about 60 to 65 degrees Fahrenheit. If air conditioning isn't an option, consider putting in a ceiling fan. The fan can also produce white noise that may help lull your child to sleep.

Keep the room adequately dark, especially in summer when daylight lasts longer. Room darkening shades and blinds can help. Don't let your child sleep with the light on, but do allow a nightlight if she's afraid of the dark.

Stifling Sound

Close your child's bedroom door, and give her a nightlight if she protests that it makes the room too dark. If she's lying there listening to the adults in the house chat, she'll have an even harder time going to sleep. A white-noise machine or CD may be useful in masking ambient sound from traffic or a poorly insulated house. Older kids might try earplugs if noise is still an issue.

Some children do better with some relaxing instrumental background music played at a low volume to lull them to sleep. Recordings of environmental sounds also work for many kids. You can find these tapes or CDs featuring forest noises (birds, leaves in the breeze), or streams and rivers, rain, and ocean waves.

So you've created a good sleep environment for your child, eliminated stimulating activities and vigorous exercise, and cut out the wrong kinds of snacks and caffeine near bedtime. If your child continues to have sleep difficulties, she should be seen by a pediatrician to rule out any medical causes for the sleep disturbance.

Chapter 16

When Your Child Stumbles

The road to a healthy weight and way of living isn't always a smooth one. It's completely normal and even expected for your child to occasionally lapse into old habits and make a poor dietary choice or skip exercise in favor of an afternoon with the Cartoon Network. The important thing is to prevent stumbles from becoming permanent falls. You can do this by making sure your child understands what causes unhealthy choices and by helping him move forward without guilt or other emotional repercussions that may paralyze his motivation and sense of self-worth.

Binges and Triggers

Your child is choosing and eating healthy foods, enjoying regular physical activity with the family, and perhaps even pursuing an individual sport or fitness routine. Then suddenly, and seemingly without warning, she goes off the deep end. She spends Saturday night on the couch with an entire bag of cookies and a bowl of ice cream covered in hot fudge.

Binges, or eating to excess, rarely occur in isolation. They are usually set off by emotional or situational triggers, an event or personal exchange that pushes the binger toward food. Sometimes the triggers are simple to figure out and to fix—a mile-high chocolate cake that Grandma brings over and insists everyone tries a slab of, or the new video game that your child plugs into right after school while he eats (and eats and eats) his snack. In these cases, minor changes (such as making gaming wait until after both snack and homework and telling Grandma to bring a fruit salad instead) provide a relatively easy preventative fix for next time.

Emotional eating is a harder habit to break. That Saturday night food-fest was probably brought on by something that happened between your child and a friend, family member, or other person in her life. If emotional pain, fear, or anxiety is a trigger to turn to the comfort of food, your child needs to recognize the link and find new and healthier avenues for coping.

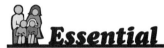 **Essential**

Don't be so protective of your child and fearful of a fitness faux pas that you restrict her unnecessarily. A bite of cheesecake or a chip or two is not a binge. As long as these indulgences are taken in moderation and your child is active and committed to healthy and balanced food choices, she should be allowed the occasional treat.

Bad Feelings: Anger, Fear, and Depression

Remember when you first taught your child how to safely cross the street? The time-tested method of "Stop, look, and listen"—stop at the corner, look both ways for cars, and listen for traffic before crossing—quickly became an ingrained habit. Emotional eating can be recognized and controlled the same way with these cues:

- **Stop.** Your child should never eat without thinking. Teach him to stop a moment, and assess the situation.
- **Look.** Your child should look within himself and at what's happening around him to find the reasons that he's eating. If he's grabbing food for any reason other than hunger, it's emotional eating.

- **Listen.** Tell your child to listen to his heart, even if what it's saying is painful. Don't smother emotional signals with food. Let feelings come to the surface.
- **Learn.** This additional fourth step is the hardest part of the process and the one where your child will need the most help. If he senses painful emotions coming his way but crosses that street to food anyway, he's going to get hurt. Staying on the curb and developing coping skills to deal with anger, fear, depression, and other bad feelings may seem the more difficult choice at first, but in the long term it will be the most effective and healthy one for your child.

Recognizing the Problem

Shame and guilt may prevent your child from sharing his problems with you. Some children are afraid of disappointing Mom or Dad. Others just want to forget a binge ever happened and move on, which is fine if they understand what motivated the initial problem and can take steps to prevent it from happening again. But even adolescents and teens may lack the introspective skills to recognize binge triggers and address them appropriately, so instead of improving the situation deteriorates further.

These clues may indicate your child is lapsing back into old behaviors:

- Food is unaccounted for, or empty food packaging is found hidden in the house.
- Weight gain occurs while your child is on a fitness program.
- Your child experiences moody, irritable, anxious, or sad behavior.
- You notice symptoms of withdrawal, with your child spending excessive time alone.

Of course, the best way to find out if your child has fallen off the fitness wagon is to simply come out and ask him. Let him know up front that you only want to help and not to judge him.

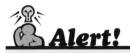

Alert!

If you think your child is frequently bingeing, it's possible she is suffering from binge-eating disorder (BED). A child with BED needs immediate treatment from a qualified mental health-care professional. Chapter 12 has more information on the diagnosis and treatment of binge-eating disorder.

After the Fall

The first order of business is to comfort your child. Make sure she understands that you aren't disappointed in her but rather are concerned about her welfare. Never ever punish or reprimand a child for falling off the fitness wagon. It's not only counterproductive, but it can also greatly erode your child's sense of self-esteem. Focus instead on how you can help her effectively deal with the lapse and move on.

Whether your child experienced a slight stumble (eating an entire bag of cookies after school) or a major face-first fall (fast food for lunch five days a week), help her to keep it in perspective. It's not the momentary lapse that matters as much as what she learns from it and how she handles future encounters with triggers for inappropriate eating.

Showing Support

Follow your child's lead to determine the best way to be supportive. Older kids may need their space to sort through things, while young children will require your help in understanding what went wrong. Younger children may also not yet have the vocabulary or insight to adequately explain how they're feeling or what might be behind their lapse. You can help by engaging them in conversation, talking about basic emotions they may be feeling (happy, sad, mad), and reassuring them of both your love and faith in their abilities.

Sitting down with a younger child and drawing pictures together is also sometimes useful. It allows small children to illustrate situations that they may not have the word power to describe verbally. Ask them to draw or paint a picture of what happened before they decided to eat too much, or suggest that they depict how they would have liked things to happen, and then talk about the artwork together.

Don't force your teen into a discussion about a lapse if she is resistant. Instead, just let her know you're there if she changes her mind, as are the other adults in her life. Suggest journaling as an option for venting, and continue to stay the course as far as providing a healthy environment free of junk food and modeling good exercise and dietary habits.

Getting Past Guilt

Kids who tie their weight and fitness goals too closely to their own sense of self-worth can be devastated over even a minor stumble. Guilt is a powerful emotion. While it may make your child work twice as hard on his fitness goals in the short term, it can also set him up for some serious self-esteem problems. Encouraging your child to feel good about himself at any size is the best way to combat the negative effects of guilt.

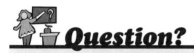 *Question?*

Should I be concerned if my son begins avoiding exercise, even if he's stuck to his food plan?

Both a nutritious diet and proper exercise are critical to your son's long-term health, so it's important to get to the bottom of his exercise aversion. Congratulate him on his commitment to healthier eating, and then ask why he's lost interest in being active. Perhaps he just hasn't found an activity he's enthusiastic about yet—an easy situation to remedy by trying out some new alternatives. If exercise is hurting him, a visit to his doctor is in order.

When Setbacks Become Roadblocks

Lapses in a diet or fitness program are not the end of the world. In fact, it's completely normal for your child to make the wrong choices occasionally. Testing her boundaries and discovering how her choices impact her life help her to develop the decision-making skills that will guide her into adulthood. Her emotional and psychological maturity are dependent on having the freedom to fall and to recover.

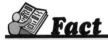 *Fact*

Binges are scary, especially if they are completely unanticipated from the parent's point of view. It's tempting to try to prevent any further food or fitness relapse by wresting control from your child and making all of her choices for her. Remind yourself that such a move will only show her you don't have faith in her decisions and will prevent her from learning from her mistakes.

Still, a bad-day binge has the potential to deter your child's progress if it isn't handled appropriately, particularly if your child ties his sense of self-worth to his appearance and weight-loss efforts. Teach your child that the key to getting past his mistakes is to learn from them, to figure out what went wrong and how to prevent it from happening again.

To keep a setback from building into a roadblock, remember these steps:

- **Stay calm.** Punishing or getting angry with your child won't accomplish anything except to make him feel inadequate and guilty, and guilt is not a healthy emotion to motivate with.
- **Offer perspective.** Stress the fact that tomorrow is another day, and while he can't change the past, he can work on the future.
- **Emphasize accomplishments.** Praise all the positive effort

your child has made toward his fitness goals to remind him of all he's achieved.

- **Keep love unconditional.** Remind your child that you love him and will always be there to support him through the good and the bad.
- **Troubleshoot together.** Offer your assistance in pinpointing the cause of the problem and strategies for future prevention.

Learning from the Fall

When you ask your child what made her eat an entire bag of chips after school, try not to get angry or frustrated if she says, "I don't know." Chances are she really doesn't know. Most adults don't recognize their own inappropriate eating patterns, so expecting a child to identify emotional eating without adult guidance is a tall order. Kids need your assistance in trying to figure out the problem and develop strategies so it doesn't occur again.

Once you've assured your child that you aren't angry and want to help, sit down and discuss how you can prevent it from happening again. It's best to do this as soon as possible so the emotions and circumstances surrounding a binge are still fresh in your child's mind. Run through these questions together to get to the root of the problem and the best way to address it:

- **How did my day start?** Did your child take time for a healthy breakfast? Did she get a good night's sleep the evening before?
- **Did I have healthy choices available for lunch and snacks?** Is your kitchen a junk-food–free zone? Are school lunch options a pass or fail?
- **Did I practice mindful eating?** Were snacks and meals eaten away from the distraction of television, video screens, and other passive entertainment that can put eating on autopilot?
- **Was I following my internal hunger cues?** Was your child snacking to satisfy hunger or because she was bored or upset about something?

- **Did I let other people's negative words or actions influence my mood?** Did someone say something that hurt your child's feelings, and if so, how did her usual coping methods fail her?

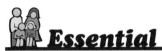

Essential

Don't fall prey to the "just this once" syndrome when it comes to allowing junk food into the house. It may be tempting to pick up those custard-stuffed chocolate éclairs for a visiting friend or relative, but bad days and binges are unpredictable, so why take the chance? You'll be doing both your child and your guest a favor by keeping your available dessert choices healthy.

The question for your child should not be, "Why am I such a screw up?" but "What can I do to keep from making that mistake again?" Sometimes those changes are simple—keep food in the kitchen, or pack a lunch instead of buying hot. In cases where triggers are tied to emotional concerns rather than logistical ones, the answers may be a little more complex.

Jamming the Triggers

Whatever strategies you set up for your child to counter binge triggers, ensure that they are constructive, action-oriented steps that address the root of the problem. Plotting revenge on someone who teases or drastically cutting calories in an effort to counter the impact of a binge don't promote healthy behaviors. Taking positive steps towards both physical and emotional fitness is the best way to keep your child's enthusiasm up and prevent a further fall.

Comfort from Friends, Not Food

If your child overeats when he's emotionally injured or drained, work with him to funnel the negative energy into positive outcomes.

Have a list of five people with whom your child feels comfortable. Encourage him to call them when he's feeling bad and needs to talk—in other words, to reach for the phone before he reaches for the refrigerator. Try to represent a good cross-section of friends and relatives so there's an ear to bend for a variety of situations. For example, he may feel comfortable talking to an aunt about family issues and a friend about a problem with a peer, but not vice-versa.

It's also possible that your child won't want to talk about what triggered a binge, at least not right away. He may be too angry or ashamed, or he may simply not have the words to adequately express his feelings right away. Channeling his anger and frustration into physical work, such as a brisk walk or bike ride, may be a good way to let him blow off steam and clear his mind for analyzing the problem.

If exercise doesn't appeal, then journaling is an excellent alternative. Spilling those complex emotions out on paper provides an opportunity to sort through them and view the situation objectively. Aside from the therapeutic value of simply venting his bad feelings, journaling also gives your child a safe place to construct theoretical scenarios for dealing with problems. Sometimes journaling about an experience offers the writer a sense of control over what seemed out of control when it happened.

 Essential

A child counselor or therapist is often a good choice for children who are unable or unwilling to talk about problems with parents or other confidants, or who seem to be having difficulty working past a lapse in their fitness program. For more on finding and working with a therapist, see Chapters 12 and 13.

Your child's journal is his emotional safety net; a place where he can talk about anything without fear of repercussion. Unless you have his explicit permission to look at it, never breach his trust by reading it. The only exception to this rule is if your child has given you reason to think that he may hurt himself or others through his words or actions.

Beating Boredom Without Food

If your child tends to eat when she's bored, work with her to compile a list of active options she can choose instead of food when she's dealing with the doldrums. Hang a copy on the refrigerator or pantry door and challenge her to complete as many as possible over the next month. Make the choices fun and varied so she can choose what suits her mood. Your list might include anything from a game of Horse at the driveway basketball hoop to planning a healthy family dinner that includes food in every color of the rainbow.

Back on Track

Once your child has experienced a fitness lapse, faced the problem, and moved forward, he'll be stronger for the experience. Praise him for his achievement.

Most importantly, if you look back, is to dwell on his victory and what he learned from it rather than on the initial stumble. It's not "Remember that time I left you alone for the afternoon and you ate all the food I bought for your brother's birthday party?" Instead, it's "I was so proud of you when you figured out what caused that setback and got right back on your food and exercise plan." If your child inspires you, let him know it. Kids, especially teens, may not always admit to caring what you think, but they do value your opinion and the pride you take in their accomplishments.

CHAPTER 17

Overweight by Age: Infants Through Preteens

Getting a stubborn toddler or preschooler to forsake his high-octane juice and Pop-Tarts for more wholesome choices may seem hopeless task. But it's well worth the effort. Food and fitness habits are formed early, so that this is actually your best window of opportunity to effectively help your overweight child. If you get your child to practice healthy lifestyle habits in her early years, by the time she hits the tumultuous teen years and decides you don't know or understand anything, she'll be better equipped to make good choices independently.

When It Isn't Just Baby Fat

It's easy to write off an overweight toddler as "solid," or having "just a little baby fat." Fortunately, if your child gets routine checkups as recommended by the American Academy of Pediatrics, your doctor should be able to detect any early weight problems or indications that your child is at risk for being overweight. Because excess weight can also be a sign of a hormonal problem or another medical condition, it's important that you don't ignore it. Book an appointment with the pediatrician even if your child's next scheduled doctor's visit isn't for several months.

Your child's doctor will not use BMI-for-age charting if your child is under age two. Instead, he will use a length-for-age and weight-for-length chart to assess growth. If your child exceeds the 95th percentile in weight for length, or her weight has suddenly increased significantly with no corresponding growth in height, she may be overweight or at risk for weight problems.

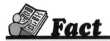 **Fact**

> From age two, BMI gradually declines until sometime between the ages of four and six, when it begins to climb again. Called "adiposity rebound," this effect is a result of increased activity in your child. A child whose BMI starts to increase before age four may be at risk for being overweight. Chapter 3 has more information on calculating body mass index (BMI).

What You Can and Can't Change

Your child's body shape is genetically influenced. If his parents are both tall and lean (called an ectomorph body type), he'll likely also be tall. If his parents are short and wide (endomorph body type), chances are he'll follow suit. An endomorph isn't destined to be fat, however. While children—like adults—can't change the shape of their bodies, they can lower their percentage of body fat and increase their lean muscle mass through proper diet and exercise.

Parents who are overweight or obese raise their child's risk for carrying weight problems into adulthood. An overweight toddler has a 40-percent chance of being obese in adulthood if he has an overweight parent, versus a 10-percent chance if his parents have normal BMIs. Parental obesity more than doubles the risk of adult obesity among all children under ten years of age, regardless of their weight. The good news is that if you join your child in her fitness efforts, both of you lower your obesity risks.

The Danger of "Diets"

Never put an infant or toddler on a weight-loss program or restrict calories or fat without guidance from your child's health-care provider. Your doctor will probably recommend a weight maintenance plan—keeping your child's weight stable (or slowing his rate of growth) to allow him to grow into his weight.

Drastically restricting caloric intake can also have the unwanted effect of causing a dietary deficiency in important vitamins and minerals that are crucial to your child's physical growth and cognitive development. For example, fat—something many parents may automatically assume should be cut from their child's diet—is actually important to infant brain and visual development.

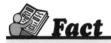 **Fact**

Infants that are breastfed exclusively usually gain weight more quickly in the first few months of life than formula-fed babies. The trend reverses at six months through one year of life, when breastfed infants weigh less than most formula-fed infants.

Hearing Hunger

Teach your infant to listen to his appetite by having leisurely feeding sessions. Do not force him to finish bottles or stay on the breast longer than he seems to want to. When he just seems to want to suck for comfort, but isn't particularly interested in food, a pacifier or even his hand may be a suitable alternative.

Your child's pediatrician will probably recommend you introduce some solid foods between four and six months of age, and the same strategy applies then. Remember that your toddler's tummy is small, and adult portions are overwhelming. If he indicates he's all finished by refusing to open his mouth or pushing away the food, don't force it. Let him self-feed as soon as he is able and interested, as this is the best way for him to eat only to his appetite.

Infancy to Preschool

Your child is in the formative years, and his attitudes towards food and exercise are just developing. He will look to you for guidance on what to eat and will also model your fitness behavior—positive or negative. Take advantage of this truly once-in-a-lifetime opportunity to set a healthy example from the very beginning.

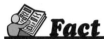 **Fact**

The American Academy of Pediatrics recommends that once children reach the age of two, they switch from regular milk to skim or low-fat. Toddlers under two need the extra fat that whole milk provides for normal growth and development.

The under-five set also gets excited about physical activity, another bonus for you as a parent. Structured movement, such as yoga poses and tumbling exercises, is fun and challenging for young children. Set it to music, and they enjoy it twice as much. Toddlers and preschoolers like to copy other kids and the instructor and to test the limits of their tiny bodies. You and your child can experience swimming, yoga, and more in classes designed for kids, or for parents and kids together.

Dietary Changes for the Demanding Toddler

For parents of willful toddlers who have already picked up some poor nutrition habits, making positive dietary changes may represent your biggest challenge. Results from the "Feeding Infants and Toddlers Study," published in the *Journal of the American Dietetic Association* in 2004, found that children under the age of three are eating more junk food and less vegetables and fruit than ever. Of over 3,000 children between the ages of four months and two years, a full third ate no fruits or veggies daily. Among those who did eat vegetables, the choice was French fries. Over 20 percent of the older children in the survey ate fries daily. FITS also found that over 60 percent of one-year-olds and over 70 percent of eighteen-month-olds ate candy or dessert daily.

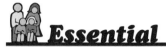

Essential

Fruit juice can be just as fattening as soda if your child drinks too much, and toddlerhood is a time when many kids get hooked on the juice bottle. Four ounces daily is the recommended limit for children between six months and a year, and kids between one and six can have four to six ounces. Older kids should be limited to eight to twelve ounces, and infants under six months should not drink juice unless a pediatrician recommends it. If your child is a juice fanatic, one way to make it last a little longer is to fill her cup halfway with juice and top it off with water.

If you recognize your child in these statistics, it isn't too late to make changes. A registered dietitian can provide menu ideas and guidance, and these tips can get you started towards healthier meals and snacks:

- **Let them be picky.** Allow your child to choose his lunch from several healthful choices. It will bolster his growing sense of independence in a positive way.
- **Shop together.** Visit the supermarket or farmer's market, and let your child help gather his favorite fruits and veggies (while avoiding the candy and cereal aisles and other danger zones).
- **Turn off the television.** Or at least stick to PBS. Many kids have no knowledge of popular sugar and fat-filled junk foods until they see them in commercials being downed by their favorite cartoon characters.
- **Offer variety.** Serving small portions of a variety of new foods

is a better approach than piling on heaping helpings of the unknown. The smaller portions are less intimidating, and with more than one option he's bound to like something on his plate.

- **Be consistent.** Most important of all, be consistent in your attitudes toward and rules surrounding food. Toddlers need to know that they have stable boundaries they can depend on, even if they don't always agree with them.
- **Push the presentation.** Modeling healthy snacks after your child's favorite not-so-healthy ones can help him make the transition. For example, if he loves potato chips, try Veggie Booty snacks, organic vegetable chips that don't have the saturated and trans fats of many brands of potato chips.

Leading by Example

Encourage your child's older siblings to try to be enthusiastic about new foods you introduce. Remind them that they're role models as far as the younger kids are concerned. Even if the older kids don't care for a dish, the idea that they're helping a little brother or sister try something new may be enough to get them to at least feign excitement over spinach.

Present a united front. If yours is a two-parent household, both Mom and Dad must be on board with house rules regarding what's allowed in the house and what isn't. You must also both make a commitment to model appropriate healthy behavior for your child. It bears repeating that a move toward fitness should involve the entire family, not just the child who is overweight or is at risk for having a weight problem.

Day-care providers or babysitters may present a special challenge. If your child is in a group setting, you probably can't control the quality of food that other children and providers have in her presence. However, you should let your concerns be known so accommodations can be made where possible. For example, if providers make a habit of dispensing candy or treats to their charges, they can do it while your child is occupied with another activity. Better yet, suggest that they replace the candy with fresh fruit for all the children. A sitter who comes to your home will probably be more accommodating about what she eats in front of your child, especially if all you have in the house is healthy food to begin with.

School-Aged to Preteens

Once your child hits the school hallways, you have the additional influences of peers, teachers, and cultural expectations to either help or hinder his fitness progress. On one hand, a regular physical education class and formal nutrition education can work in your favor. On the other, he may befriend other kids who sit down with a bag of chips and a video game after school—exactly what you're steering him away from.

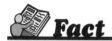 **Fact**

While your child may be looking more and more to his peers as he decides what to dress and how to act, you still hold substantial influence—even into the preteen years. Continue to model good behavior, even when you think your child isn't paying attention. He will notice, especially if you adopt a "Do as I say, *and* as I do" policy towards fitness and food.

Don't take it for granted that your child gets adequate exercise and balanced meals at school. Educate yourself about the quality of the school lunch program and the curriculum used in phys ed and nutrition education. Talk to the principal and teachers, and attend parent-teacher organization meetings. If you have concerns about how food and fitness programs are conducted, attend your local school-board meeting and let your views be known. Chapter 19 has more information on regulations surrounding nutrition and phys ed in the schools and how you can help shape policy at your child's school.

As your child hits the magic double-digits in age, she'll want more independence, but she may not be mature enough yet to handle it. Preteens live in the moment and rarely understand the long-term consequences of their choices. This can have implications on the way you motivate them into following a fitness routine. Telling your preteen son that daily exercise will lower his risk of heart disease won't exactly light a fire under him. However, telling him that it will increase his endurance for the rafting trip he's been begging to join will probably get him moving.

When you focus on the short-term payoff as a motivator, make sure you don't fall into the trap of stressing appearance rather than overall health and a sense of well-being. Don't tell your daughter she needs to work out to fit into the dress she wants for the fifth-grade dance. Ask her instead if she'd like to take some Jazzercise or dance classes so she can feel good dancing the night away.

Of course, the preteen years can also bring hormonal and physical changes that can make a weight problem even more complicated. This is especially the case for girls, who may be gaining weight as a result of early puberty or prepuberty. Chapter 18 discusses the impact of puberty on body weight and how it can affect the overweight child.

Peer Power

Peer influence grows in importance throughout the school years. By the time kids reach middle school, what their friends do and what others think of them is often a central concern in their lives. Developmentally, this is a normal place for your child to be, as she begins to seek out independence from her parents. Yet it can also be a maddening time for Mom and Dad as a child turns towards her peers, and away from you, for direction in her life. Peer pressure is frequently positive, and it can guide your child towards healthy interests and attitudes. But if friends are exerting negative influences or your child is being victimized by peers at school, she needs your guidance (whether she knows it or not).

Enlisting Allies

When your child hangs out with kids who seem to eat everything and do nothing (at least in a physical sense), it can be a difficult task to get him motivated to exercise in his free time. While he needs the autonomy to pick his own friends, it doesn't hurt to nurture potential new peer relationships that may share fitness interests. If he's interested and agreeable, group sports, dance, or exercise instruction can be good venues for finding new friends who are enthusiastic about the same activities. Take him to the skating rink, the swimming pool, and other places where kids get active.

Widening your child's circle of friends doesn't mean she has to "get rid of" her old buddies. And who knows? As she gains enthusiasm for physical activities, her passion may motivate them to get moving, too.

Taunts and Teases

Kids who feel good about themselves at any weight are typically more resilient to any teasing from peers about their size. When the teaser sees he isn't getting the intended reaction of anger or tears, he'll probably move on. If he doesn't, strong friendships with loyal friends who stick up for your child can take the sting out of taunts and teases from others. Continue to nurture those positive relationships by making your child's friends welcome in your home.

Building the Skills for Self-Improvement

A child with confidence in her abilities and who feels good about the person she is likely to have an easier time meeting the challenge of a new fitness program than a child with low self-esteem. Helping your child to recognize her inherent value is just as important, if not more so, than controlling her weight. Weight loss is not a panacea for other problems in her life. She can't be happy with the way she feels and looks until she's happy about who she is.

You can help your young child build faith in herself and her abilities by allowing her to make decisions on her own and then backing those choices. Even if it's just whether to wear the red shirt or the green one, free choice is a good exercise in helping your child realize that her decisions have value.

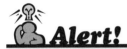

Alert!

Don't undermine your child's blossoming independence by letting her make a choice and then telling her it's a bad one. As long as her choices don't compromise her safety, they don't infringe on the rights of others, and are reasonable, let them stand. Does it really matter if she chooses a polka-dotted shirt and plaid pants? As a wise mother once said, choose your battles and forget the rest.

Expose your child to new places, people, and experiences. When she's encouraged to take social risks, she gains confidence in her communication and relationship skills. It's also a good practice to give her age-appropriate responsibilities. Even toddlers can pick up their toys or fill the pet's food and water bowl. Completing tasks and meeting responsibilities gives your child a sense of achievement and builds further self-reliance. Once a child feels capable, trusted, and valued, she will be empowered to meet the fitness goals ahead of her.

CHAPTER 18

Overweight by Age: Adolescence Through Young Adult

The emerging adolescent knows everything (and what he doesn't know, his friends do). While he recognizes that bad things do happen, he usually only considers them happening to others. These two character traits can make it difficult to have a positive influence on your child's weight-loss efforts. As adolescents mature into young adults, their world-view becomes less egocentric. They'll once again become appreciative of their parents' knowledge and experience (believe it or not). Until then, continue to support them in their physical and psychological development and weight-loss efforts.

Puberty and Weight

The teen years are inherently tough. The addition of a weight problem to the physical and emotional changes already in store for your child with puberty makes these years that much tougher. On average, puberty starts between ages eight to thirteen in girls and ages nine to fourteen in boys. When girls reach puberty, they gain body fat in the breasts and hips, while boys develop more muscle mass. Both result in weight gain, and this transformation can make an already overweight child feel even more self-conscious. Make sure your child is aware that the changes to her body are completely normal and that everyone goes through them at some point in their lives.

Changes in hormone levels can also cause mood swings and emotional outbursts in your child, which can affect both her drive and attitude towards exercise and healthy behaviors. Usually these temporary mood swings don't stick around long enough to be a major detriment to your child's fitness program. But do be aware of the signs and symptoms of depression in case it's more than just moodiness.

Growth Spurts

Once a child reaches the end of his growth spurt of puberty, he will have reached his full adult height, with no further opportunity for "growing into" his weight. This occurs slightly later in boys than in girls, who usually reach adult height about two years after their first period. Just how tall your child gets is determined largely by the height of his parents; there are several formulas to predict adult height, but none is completely foolproof.

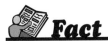 **Fact**

A landmark 1997 Virginia Commonwealth University study of 17,000 girls found that those who were overweight had an earlier onset of puberty. Several studies since then have indicated an association between the hormone leptin, weight problems, and the early onset of puberty in girls.

Two simple ways to get an idea of your child's ultimate height are the two-years-times-two method and the genetic potential formula. The two-years-times-two method is just that—take your child's height at two years old and double it. To compute your child's predicted height using genetic potential, add Mom's and Dad's heights together, divide by two, and then subtract 2.5 inches for girls or add 2.5 inches for boys.

Social Issues

Your teenager probably spends more time with his peers now than he has, or will, at any other point in his life. The people he hangs around with and what he chooses to do with the time can have a major impact on his weight-control success and motivation.

When you live in a town with few places for young people to get together, kids are often forced to gather at malls, fast-food restaurants, and pizza places, locations where your overweight teen faces even more temptation and pressure. Even the movies can be a food trap. (For more on helping your child face the concession stand, see Chapter 14.) Having an open-door policy for your teen's friends—and giving them some privacy and space when they do hang out at your home—can minimize the time they spend at the local McDonald's. It also allows you to get to know your child's circle of friends, something not all parents have the opportunity or take the time to do.

If there are more active venues in your town for teens to frequent, such as skateboarding parks and dance clubs, offer transportation and/or entrance fees to encourage these options. Once your teen starts driving, the logistical constraints on his social life will become less of a concern. However, if he's biked or walked everywhere until earning his license, it will be important for him to realize that he's losing that form of exercise and should replace it with another activity.

Dating

Like any teen with a pulse, your child is now interested in members of the opposite sex as more than friends. What do you do when her attentions aren't reciprocated, or worse, when she's shunned because of her size?

Heavy kids may not get invited to dances or asked to the movies as frequently as their thinner peers. It's unfair, but it's reality. Teenaged girls and boys can be superficial, and they won't always look past the weight to see the beautiful kid within. Considering the media influences facing these kids, it isn't surprising.

What You Should Do

As a parent, you can lessen the pain a little by encouraging your child to enjoy her friends. Tell her that when the right time and person comes along, a dating relationship will happen naturally. If there's a special dance or a couples' event like the prom that your teen hasn't been invited to, you might offer to spring for a get-together at your house for other kids who aren't going. You might also plan a special family trip somewhere adventurous.

Continue to schedule regular fun fitness activities during family time. There's probably less of it now that your child has reached the teen years, but a once-weekly time set aside for family only is important to keeping your kids grounded, maintaining open lines of communication, and reaching your fitness goals. Make attendance mandatory for both you and your kids.

What You Shouldn't Do

Never tell your child anything like this: "If you lose a few pounds, the boys will see how pretty you are." If your teen says, "Steve will never ask me out because I'm ugly," then counter with, "Then Steve must not know you very well." Remind your daughter that the best and most fulfilling relationships are based not on dress size but on attraction to kindness, sense of humor, and other personality attributes. Inner beauty sounds cliché and your teen may roll her eyes at you, but it's true. If appropriate, you may even want to explain the qualities that made you fall in love with your spouse. You might engage your daughter in a discussion about why she's feeling ugly and how your family can further support her weight-loss efforts in the context of improving her health, not her dating life.

Self-Image

The teen years are full of self-doubt for even the most confident kids, as teens pull away from the family and exercise their growing autonomy. Are they wearing the right clothes? Will their friends like their new haircut? Gaining peer acceptance is a big priority, and when it doesn't happen, a teen's self-confidence can take a serious hit. Overweight teens may be particularly susceptible to self-doubt because they don't fit the mold of physical beauty that the media has been selling for so long. In addition, they may start to feel even more conscious of their appearance as puberty strikes and their bodies change.

But when the role models that surround them are positive, and they have a solid sense of who they are and what qualities your family values, they can get through these turbulent times with minimal damage to their self-esteem.

 Essential

Volunteering is a great way to build your child's sense of self-esteem while reinforcing the importance of assistance, empathy, and kindness towards others. When she sees how much the people she works with appreciate her help, she will have a greater sense of her value and place in the world. Senior centers, hospitals, and animal shelters are just a few places that appreciate responsible teen volunteers. Teens who like to work with kids can also join a mentoring program.

Doing Your Part

Reinforce the good qualities you see your teen demonstrate by expressing your pride and appreciation. Your teen may be embarrassed by your praise if it's given in front of others, but it's still important for him to hear it. Wait until the two of you are alone, and let him know why you're impressed: "It was really thoughtful of you to let your little sister go to the movies with you and your friends. I know you would've rather left her at home, but it meant a lot to her and to me that you recognized how excited she was about it."

As a parent, you should continue to set a good example. Though it may not always seem like your child is paying attention, he is. Don't talk about yourself negatively or behave in a way you wouldn't want to see your teen behaving. Everyone shows a bad side once in a while—think about the last time someone cut you off on the freeway—but try not to let it come out in front of your child. When you do lose it in front of your teen, be sure to apologize. Later, when you've cooled off, explain why your behavior was wrong. Above all, don't speak negatively about others when your child is within earshot. (Better yet, try to frame all of your comments about others in a positive way, regardless of who's listening.) If your teen has had the experience of being cut down by a peer, to hear a parent exhibit the same behavior will just validate the behavior and the message.

"Fitting In" When You Look Different

Being part of the crowd and feeling accepted by peers are important to teens. Those with weight problems may feel as though they stick out like a sore thumb. Remind your child that while he may not have the same body type as his peers, he shares many of the same interests, attitudes, and dreams for the future. Encourage him to get more involved in those areas of interest and value his friendships there.

Let your child have autonomy when it comes to buying clothes and accessories. This is a particularly important issue for style-conscious teenage girls. Your teen's larger size requirements may mean she can't find clothing in many of the stores where her friends shop. Don't force her to shop in the women's department or at a "full-figured" store that caters to adults. She'll only feel even more self-conscious about looking different than her peers.

Some junior departments are starting to offer plus-sized offerings, but it's still the exception rather than the rule. Fortunately, there are growing style options in both online and brick-and-mortar stores. For example, Torrid, a California-based store with shops nationwide, offers trendy clothes in sizes 12 to 26 for teens and young adult women. Appendix B has more shopping resources for plus-sized teens.

Advertising and Media Messages

The American Psychological Association's task force on advertising and children found that advertisers spend over $12 billion annually on messages targeting youth. Teens are an important part of the youth demographic. They are developing brand awareness and spending habits that will carry over into adulthood. Many have jobs or receive other disposable income from their parents that product manufacturers and the entertainment industry are eager to get a cut of. Unfortunately, the media messages these companies use to attract teens aren't always the healthiest.

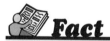 *Fact*

In its policy statement on Media Education, the American Academy of Pediatrics' Committee on Public Education recommends that state and federal government "explore mandating and funding universal media education programs with demonstrated effectiveness in American schools." Appendix B has more media literacy resources that may help you get a program started in your child's school.

Kids are inundated with advertisements for sugar and fat-filled foods, yet the models and actors used to sell it look as if they've never eaten a bite of junk food themselves. The National Institute on Media and the Family reports that the average child sees over 10,000 television ads annually for food. Just the act of sitting and watching television can stimulate mindless snacking, and the barrage of food images doesn't help.

Find out if your child's junior or high school offers media literacy curriculum in any courses, such as journalism, and encourage your child to take the class. Most teens will probably be intrigued by the concept. Media literacy teaches kids to evaluate messages with a critical eye, to examine economic, social, and political motivations and manipulations in the images they see, and to recognize more subtle forms of advertising like product placements in television and movies.

Media Beauty Is Only Skin Deep

As your teen becomes immersed in the messages popular culture is sending her via movies, television, magazines, music, and other mediums, she may be more vulnerable to low self-esteem and a poor self-image.

A study cosponsored by Children Now and the Kaiser Family Foundation found that the physical beauty of women and girls is a major theme in broadcast media. In movies, 58 percent of female characters received comments on their appearance, compared to only 24 percent of male characters. The study also found that across all print and broadcast media, between 26 and 46 percent of women are thin (for men, the numbers were significantly lower—between 4 and 16 percent). Among magazines specifically targeted to teenage girls, over a third of the articles were focused on appearance and physical beauty. The overall message seems to be how girls look is more important than who they are and that thin is definitely in.

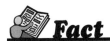 **Fact**

Adolescent girls who are overweight (or believe they are overweight) are 50 percent more likely to start smoking as a weight-control tool than those who perceive their body weight as normal or low.

Again, media literacy education can help your teen recognize the reality behind those incredibly beautiful shots of slim models in her favorite magazines. She'll learn about media techniques such as airbrushing and digital manipulation of photos that erase physical imperfections on the page and screen. She should also understand what the average measurements, weights, and height are of a real American woman or teen versus the typical model.

Pills and Procedures

Obese teens are increasingly turning to surgery and drugs for weight loss. While these options may be appropriate for some obese adolescents who face serious weight-related health complications, they are not a first-line treatment. Neither surgery nor medication should ever be employed before nutritional and exercise changes have been given an adequate time to work. In addition, drugs and surgery may be perceived as a quick fix to a problem that requires long-term strategies to overcome. In the end, using these methods is a decision to be made on a case-by-case basis with your teen and your doctor.

Weight-Loss Drugs

Prescription medications Meridia (sibutramine, from Abbott Laboratories) and Xenical (orlistat, from Roche Pharmaceuticals) have shown some effectiveness in treating teen obesity. Orlistat works by blocking fat absorption, and sibutramine suppresses appetite. Orlistat received FDA market clearance for use by obese teens in late 2003. The drug does have some potential side effects, including possible gas and stool leakage. It can also impair the absorption of some fat-soluble vitamins, requiring daily multivitamin supplementation.

The FDA has not cleared Meridia for use by teens, but clinical studies have demonstrated its effectiveness in this population. However, Meridia has come under fire by consumer watchdog group Public Citizen, which claims that the drug may be linked to heart-disease deaths. Both the manufacturer (Abbott Labs) and the American Obesity Association deny that claim, and to date there is no published clinical evidence supporting it.

Drug therapy is usually only recommended for those teens who are significantly overweight and who have been unsuccessful in losing weight via lifestyle changes. It's important that they keep up those lifestyle changes, however. A weight-loss drug is just a temporary aid in fighting fat, and one that can't work alone indefinitely.

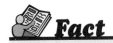 **Fact**

> According to a U.S. Department of Health and Human Services–sponsored study in the *Archives of Pediatrics & Adolescent Medicine*, U.S. teenagers have a higher likelihood of being overweight than teens from fourteen other industrialized nations: Austria, the Czech Republic, Denmark, Flemish Belgium, Finland, France, Germany, Greece, Lithuania, Ireland, Israel, Portugal, Slovakia, and Sweden.

Gastric Bypass

A growing number of teens are undergoing gastric-bypass, or bariatric, surgery. This invasive procedure involves reducing the size of the stomach so that it only accommodates a small portion of food. While it can facilitate dramatic weight loss, it is a permanent and major lifestyle change and should not be considered lightly. Teens considering bariatric surgery should be carefully screened for both their physical and psychological readiness for the procedure.

After the surgery, teens must take vitamins and minerals (particularly calcium carbonate, to prevent osteoporosis, and iron supplements) for the rest of their lives. If they attempt to eat more than their stomach will accommodate (less than one cup) or have foods high in fat or sugar, they experience severe gastrointestinal distress and nausea. They must also drink small amounts of water and sugar-free beverages throughout the day to prevent dehydration.

The International Pediatric Endosurgery Group (IPEG) has set the following guidelines for selecting adolescent candidates for bariatric surgery:

- Candidate must have a BMI of 40 or higher with serious medical co-morbidities (such as Type 2 diabetes or obstructive sleep apnea), **OR**
- Candidate must have a BMI of 50 or higher with minor medical co-morbidities (such as hypertension, high cholesterol).

- Candidate must also meet all following criteria:
  - Have reached (or nearly reached) full adult height
  - Be capable of following postoperative care and nutrition guidelines
  - Be willing to undergo a psychological examination
  - Have undergone a minimum of six months of conventional weight management attempts (diet and exercise) with poor results
  - Agree to not become pregnant for a year after the surgery

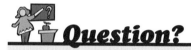

Question?

How can I change the eating habits of my sixteen-year-old when I'm not cooking for her?
Teach her to cook! She may be eating junk simply because she doesn't have the culinary skills to make a healthy meal. You might even find a local cooking class in a cuisine she particularly enjoys to spice things up. Whatever you select, make sure the curriculum is slanted towards healthy cooking methods and foods.

Transition to Adult Weight Issues

Teens with weight problems often grow into adults with weight problems. A study of young adults in Washington State examined their childhood and parental height and weight records. Results showed that obese teens have more than a 50-percent chance of remaining obese into adulthood, and those odds increase to as much as 80 percent if a parent is also obese. That does *not* mean that your teen is destined to remain overweight. Start working with your family to control weight. Break unhealthy habits now, and your child can start on the path to fitness while she is still at home and surrounded by supportive family.

College-Bound

If your teen will be headed off to college soon or is looking at her options, it's a good idea to plan to get a support system in place to help her continue her fitness routine once she's there. At college, teens may be completely without parental supervision for the first time in their lives, and you want her to be prepared for the challenges she'll face. When you visit schools, find out what the food service is like and what meal plan options are available. Investigate the fitness facilities, and equip her to face and conquer the famed "freshman fifteen."

Although clinical studies have disagreed on whether the college freshman fifteen-pound weight gain is a real phenomenon, most are in agreement that there are some real fitness pitfalls awaiting new college students. These include the following:

- **Study load.** College means lots of time spent sitting and hitting the books. Encourage your child to break it up a bit with occasional walks and exercise intermissions—it will benefit her mind as well as her body.
- **Coin-operated calories.** From the student union to the dorms, vending machines are everywhere and tempting to time-starved students. Invest in a mini-fridge and microwave for your teen's dorm room so she can stock up on alternatives to the usual vending machine fare.
- **Seconds, thirds, and fourths.** Food service programs that offer all-you-can-eat dining add temptation. Make sure your teen is educated about portion control and wise food choices before she heads off to school.
- **Parties.** Alcohol can pack on the pounds. Talk to your child about drinking responsibly, for her health as well as for her safety.

Health and Disease Risks

The sooner you begin working with your teen and your family to get healthy, the sooner he cuts his risk for adult health problems like Type 2 diabetes, cardiovascular disease, high cholesterol levels, and hypertension (high blood pressure). If he already has some of these problems, along with any other common ailments of obese teens, such as obstructive sleep apnea and asthma, dropping pounds will not only relieve symptoms and make him feel more energetic, it may also save his life.

CHAPTER 19

Educating the Schools: Healthy Bodies, Healthy Minds

Outside of your home, school is the place where your child spends most of her time. Therefore, it's essential that her educators share your vision for healthy food and fitness goals. You may just assume that schools offer the most nutritious menu options and promote daily physical exercise by virtue of their role as child nurturers and caretakers. However, that isn't always the case. Fortunately, parent input can help change both health curriculum and meal choices for the better.

Phys Ed: A Lost Opportunity?

Physical education class is probably the single best opportunity your child has to develop a passion for exercise; gain physical strength, agility, and athletic skill; and learn the cerebral side of physical activity, such as sportsmanship and strategy. Why then do so many kids, particularly overweight kids, avoid the locker room like the plague?

Sometimes it's embarrassment at what a child perceives as his lack of athletic skills or endurance. Other times a child is intimidated by his peers or by the curriculum or uninspired by the activity choices he has been given. To add even further complexity to the situation, many physical education programs find themselves faced with program cuts and dwindling resources as school districts look for ways to meet budget demands. So an already limited phys ed program may be restricted even further.

If your child seems lukewarm about his phys ed program, consider these reasons his school's program may be missing the mark:

- **Reduced number of classes.** If funding is at a premium at your child's school, and physical education guidelines are not mandated by the district or state board of education, she may get a limited amount of physical education instruction each week, if any.
- **Expensive equipment.** Your child's teacher may also be limited in the variety of activities he offers to your child, based on what the school has budgeted for equipment and safety gear.
- **Monotony.** Can your child count on one of the same four activities every time she suits up for gym class? A phys ed teacher who's stuck in a rut won't do much to inspire athleticism in your child.
- **One size fits all.** Does your child's instructor plan activities that both the most advanced and the least accomplished athletes can participate in? A physical education curriculum that isn't scalable to different skill levels will probably be extremely frustrating to your child.
- **Intimidation.** If the jocks in the class dominate a game or get upset with players who aren't as adept at a sport as they are, your child won't be too wild about participating.

Expanding Options

When financial considerations have limited your child's PE program, there are ways to help. Speak with the parent-teacher organization about the possibility of a fundraising drive for new gym equipment. Give some of your own time for extracurricular activities, such as a walking club after school or during recess. Suggest that your school get involved in national nonprofit fundraising events like the American Diabetes Association's Walk for Diabetes or the American Heart Association's Jump Rope for Heart.

Recruiting Volunteers

You can also talk to the phys ed teachers or district directors about their interest in using volunteers from the community to expand their program. There may be some insurance and liability issues to address, but if those can be overcome, a volunteer program can add a whole spectrum of new and exciting fitness activities to a school's physical education curriculum.

Recruit instructors from the local gym or YMCA to come in and volunteer their time to teach yoga, kickboxing, and a variety of other activities. They will benefit from free advertising, an opportunity to recruit new students (and their parents) into their private classes, and the knowledge that they've helped their community. If recruitment efforts are moving slowly, talk with the local newspaper about your efforts. They may consider running a feature on the program or at the least running a free ad in their community section to recruit more instructors.

Use Your Voting Power

The most important thing you can do to ensure the phys ed program at your child's school continues to get the support it deserves is to stay on top of what is happening at the school, the district, and at the state level. Communicate your concerns to the school principal. Talk to your child's phys ed teacher or the school phys ed director, if there is one, about how parents and the district can better support their goals for the program. Attend school-board meetings, and write or call your state representative about educational legislation that influences the quantity and quality of physical activity your child gets at school.

This isn't always an easy task, and legislation that may on the surface have nothing to do with physical education can turn out to make a substantial difference. For example, a mandate to extend the number of hours devoted to academic curriculum may cause some principals to reduce time spent on physical education and recess and redirect those hours towards academics so they don't have to alter the length of the school day. Unless you're working for the school district or are in government, it's impossible to keep up on all developments, but you can let your elected officials know that you value the importance of a healthy level of daily activity at school. Encourage your friends and neighbors to do the same so your representatives will act in their constituents' best interests.

 Essential

Ask your school principal to make inexpensive equipment such as jump ropes and playground balls available to kids at recess so they can have a variety of fun and physical activities to engage in aside from the usual playground equipment.

Slimming Down the Lunch Line

As a parent, you may just take the nutritional value of your child's school lunch offerings as a given. After all, public schools and private schools that receive any form of federal funding must be providing meals that are nutritionally balanced and in line with the USDA food pyramid, right?

Well, not exactly. While the USDA's Food and Nutrition Service (FNS) does regulate the school lunch program, there are no guarantees that today's cafeteria special will meet recommended daily allowances of nutrients and fall within acceptable caloric and fat standards. Menu planning standards required by the FNS do suggest nutritional guidelines and recommended daily allowances (RDAs), but they fail to make schools financially or legally accountable for meeting anything but the loosest requirements.

The USDA is also charged with ensuring the financial well-being of American farmers, which further complicates the school nutrition picture. The majority of federally subsidized surplus commodities—those foods like cheese and beef that the government has promised to purchase from farmers to keep market prices where they should be—are donated to the school lunch program. Some critics have charged that this arrangement leads to an excess of fat and calories on the school lunch menu.

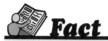

Fact

In addition to the federal school lunch program, the FNS also administers a school breakfast program and an after-school snack program. Some studies have shown a link between weight problems and skipping breakfast. Research published in 2003 in the *American Journal of Epidemiology* found that breakfast-skippers were 4.5 times more likely to be overweight.

Food-Based Versus Nutrient-Standard Menu Planning

Under the USDA's School Meals Initiative for Healthy Children, school lunch programs are allowed to operate under one of two menu planning strategies: food-based menu planning or nutrient-standard menu planning. The former is more widely used and has been in place since the school lunch program was created in 1946. The latter is newer. It uses computer software to analyze the specific nutrient content of foods offered and ensure that when averaged over a school week, the meals offered on the lunch menu meet one-third of the RDA for specific nutrients and calories based on age and/or grade.

With food-based menu planning, certain food types (such as meats or grains and breads) have to be served up in specific quantities at a meal. Those food types and quantities follow the USDA food pyramid. The main shortcoming of this type of planning is that it does not offer any inherent safeguards to ensure that unhealthy (like saturated fat) and healthy (such as calcium) nutrients are within recommended limits. In other words, a food-based menu could follow the pyramid to the letter and be fat-heavy and nutrient-poor, or exceed recommended calorie allowances for age.

The USDA does suggest that meal planners using the food-based method keep calories to one-third of the daily RDA for each age group served, limit total fat to 30 percent of calories and saturated fat to 10 percent, and try to meet RDA guidelines for other key nutrients. However, there are no requirements to use nutritional analysis to achieve this and no penalties for not meeting these requirements. Furthermore, these suggested nutritional guidelines are based not on each specific meal, but rather on a week's worth of averaged menus.

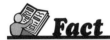 **Fact**

While national monitoring of school lunch menu-planning is not in place, the FNS does require that state agencies administer and periodically review the school lunch program. This task is usually assigned to the state department of education, although it may occasionally be handled by the state's department of health and human services or agriculture. For more information on what government entity administers your school lunch program, see the FNS directory on the Web at ✐*www.fns.usda.gov.*

For these reasons, it's important to ask your school's food service director what menu-planning system the school uses. Push for the school to do actual nutritional analysis of menus whenever possible. If the information is available, there's no reason that nutrient values can't be printed on the monthly school menus that are sent home with your child.

Providing Nutritional Analysis

The USDA requires that all nutritional analysis of foods for school lunch programs be done using approved software that contains the USDA child nutrition database, or CN. The CN database contains nutritional values for common school lunch and breakfast items and for commodities schools frequently receive.

If your child's school performs nutritional analysis of menus, the USDA requires it to assess the amount of fat (total and saturated), calories, calcium, iron, protein, vitamin A, and vitamin C. The standard amounts of each of these nutrients, excluding fat, vary by either age group or grade (depending on the type of calculation the school is using). Total fat should calculate to no more than 30 percent of calories, and of that 30 percent, no more than 10 percent of calories should be from saturated fat. Unfortunately, there are no limits or standards on cholesterol and sodium other than a nonspecific mandate to try and reduce them while increasing fiber content.

Fast Food Versus Whole Food Choices

Many schools are turning to for-profit à la carte items from fast-food franchises and other vendors to supplement their budgets. Contracts for brand-name pizzas, burgers, and fries—items in high demand for which kids with disposable income are willing to pay a premium—bring in big bucks for school programs. Federal school-lunch nutrition guidelines, however imperfect they are, don't even apply to these foods because they aren't considered reimbursable (that is, part of the free or reduced-cost FNS school lunch program).

What's a parent to do? As an initial step, you can send a healthy and appealing lunch to school with your child so he isn't tempted to spend his money on cafeteria fast food. Then, you can talk with school officials about your concerns with the high-fat fare. Ask if the vendor might be able to offer some more balanced choices with his à la carte offerings. If you can't get any satisfaction, take your argument higher—to your state senators and representatives. Many lawmakers are starting to take legislative action on limiting access to unhealthy food in school.

Vending Machines

Do you have a vending machine at your office or place of business that seems to call your name when lunchtime approaches? Go and take a look at what snacks and treats are nestled amongst the rotating coils. Is there anything even remotely healthy—such as trail mix, dried fruit, sunflower seeds, or whole-wheat crackers? Chances are at least 80 percent of the snacks are candy, chips, and other assorted junk foods. And odds are that the vending machines in your child's school are even worse.

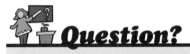

Question?

Is it true that the principal of a school has no control over the food choices offered in the cafeteria?

Yes and no—he may not create the menus, but he should be able to convey your concerns to those who can. If he isn't being helpful, call the school district and ask who directs the food-service program. That is probably your best starting point for airing your concerns. If the district outsources menu planning to a private company, consider bringing up the issue at the next school-board meeting.

Improving the Options

Vending machine foods, particularly the nonrefrigerated variety, are frequently chock-full of preservatives that extend their shelf life. That doesn't mean that vending machines are completely hopeless. Ask your school or school district to request that snack vendors offer healthier choices. Even if the school has a long-term contract with a vending company, they should be able to work together to come up with acceptable alternatives.

Snack-sized packages of raisins, granola or oat bars, applesauce cups, whole-wheat pretzels, and air-popped popcorn are just a few healthy vending machine ideas. Beverage machines can hold low-fat and skim milk, a variety of flavored and plain bottled waters, and 100-percent fruit juices.

Another short-term fix is to turn the machines off at certain times of the day. The FNS requires that schools participating in the National

School Lunch Program limit access to vending machines during all school-lunch periods. Make sure your child's school is adhering to that policy. That doesn't stop students from accessing the vending machines during other times of day, but it's a step in the right direction.

Sayonara, Soda

Sometime over the past several decades, soda has become a ubiquitous "kid" drink, and Coke and Pepsi machines have sprung up in school cafeterias and hallways nationwide. But with the fattening of America's youth and adults and the revelation of several clinical studies that have found a definite link between excessive soda and soft-drink consumption and childhood weight problems, the drink has been demonized. And not without good reason—one can of regular Coke has 97 calories and 27 grams of sugar in a mere eight ounces, or two-thirds of a can. Pepsi weighs in at 100 calories and 27 grams of sugar.

But as school departments and lawmakers move to push soda out of the schools, it's important for them to realize that soda isn't the only problem. Many "fruit drinks" offer little juice and lots of sugar as well. Even too many sports drinks, when they're not used primarily as a rehydrating beverage during sports or strenuous physical activity, can pack on the pounds. Making low-fat milk, diet sodas, bottled water, and low- or no-sugar-added teas and pure fruit juices available for thirsty kids is the best choice.

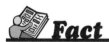 **Fact**

Some states have drafted or passed legislation that forbids or limits the sale of soda and unhealthful snacks, despite the financial attraction of vending deals. Until the sale of foods of "limited nutritional value" in schools was restricted by the Texas agriculture commissioner in 2003, school soda vending-machine contracts were pumping an extra $54 million annually into the Texas school system alone.

Avoiding Mixed Messages

Schools often offer healthy choices for meals and then push unhealthy options outside the cafeteria. Frequently, when poor food choices are found in or around school, it's because of financial incentives that budget-strapped schools find hard to pass up. Soda and vending companies can offer lucrative donations and sponsorships in exchange for the freedom to place their products in front of kids. Fundraising organizations push candy as a high-margin product for schoolchildren to sell. Concession stands at high-school football games serve up fried foods and candy without offering other healthier options, perhaps not quite as profitable, like sandwich wraps and fresh fruits. Money for updated facilities, better educational and extracurricular programs, and academic supplies is important, but the price is too dear if it's costing children their health and undermining school nutrition and phys ed policies.

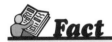 *Fact*

The School Health Policies and Program Study (2000; U.S. CDC) determined that over 98 percent of high schools have vending machines or other purchase points outside of the cafeteria where students buy food and drinks, and that most available foods were high in sugar, sodium, and fats.

Fundraisers

Preaching good nutrition and then telling children to go sell as much candy as possible for the good of the school sends a very mixed message to your child about promoting healthy behavior. Encourage your school administrators and parent-teacher association to avoid fundraisers that push fat- and sugar-rich, nutrient-poor foods. If they insist on selling candy, ask that they ban fundraising candy sales from the school building itself or from taking place during school hours to discourage kids from buying and eating throughout the day.

Appropriate Alternatives

A good alternative to the typical candy and wrapping-paper fundraising options may be to involve the school in partnering with local farmers, orchards, or produce wholesalers and creating their own farmers' market at the school. This can be a great learning experience for kids of all ages. It would give them the chance to visit the farm, learn more about where fresh fruits and vegetables come from, and perhaps even help out during planting and harvesting season in exchange for free produce to sell.

Health and Nutrition Education

According to the U.S. CDC, an estimated 90 percent of all U.S. school districts require a nutritional education component to their health curriculum. Does your child's school curriculum include age-appropriate units on nutrition and its importance to health and disease prevention? Does it address the importance of an active lifestyle in health maintenance? Requirements for health education vary by state and district policy. Check with your school district or state department of education to determine what the standards are.

Nutrition curriculum is often tied into the food service offerings at a school or district. The FNS offers a variety of educational materials for teachers and students. It's always good policy to practice what you preach, so if the food your child is faced with in the cafeteria doesn't meet the standards prescribed in the nutrition education she's receiving, talk to her teacher or principal about it.

Peer Sensitivity Training

Beyond promoting physical health through better physical education programs and more nutritious lunch menus, it's important that your child's school also serve his emotional needs. If your child or any other student is being teased or terrorized by peers because of weight, and school officials haven't been able to intervene effectively, peer-sensitivity training for the class or student body may be an appropriate suggestion. A guidance counselor may be able to conduct the training, or the school can hire an outside consultant with the appropriate experience and credentials.

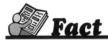

A peer-mediation program is different from peer-sensitivity training, but it may also be useful if your child is having problems at school. Peer mediators are students who are trained to peacefully resolve conflicts between children by clarifying the facts of the situation and helping the participants solve problems and reach a solution. They teach other children how to listen to each other and communicate more effectively.

The reasons kids tease and bully are complex and varied. Sometimes it's attention-seeking behavior. At other times, a child may mimic what he's learned from adults and siblings in his life. Peer-sensitivity training focuses on promoting a sense of understanding and empathy toward others who are different in appearance, abilities, or beliefs. It also emphasizes a basic code of conduct of kindness to others, no matter who they are, and a structured discipline system for those who break that code. A workshop or school assembly on peer sensitivity will benefit not just your son or daughter but every child and teacher who participates.

CHAPTER 20

Weight Loss and Special Dietary Needs

Sometimes weight loss efforts are hampered by food allergies and other chronic health conditions. Your family's cultural heritage and personal belief system can also play a part in what foods and dishes you allow into your household and the composition of your daily diet. The good news is that no matter what your dietary requirements, there's virtually always room for making healthy adjustments to the family diet.

Vegetarianism and Weight Control

Overall, studies have shown that most vegetarians are leaner and have lower total cholesterol levels than their meat-eating counterparts. While it certainly would be nice if a diet heavy in fruits and vegetables were a guaranteed ticket to perfect fitness, the truth is that it is possible for vegetarians, vegans included, to be overweight.

If your family lives a vegetarian lifestyle and your child has a weight problem, take a good look at the kinds of foods your child is consuming and the types of activities she is participating in on a daily basis. Is she getting her share of daily exercise? Are fats and sweets used sparingly? Keeping a food and fitness journal is the best way to pinpoint any problems.

Nutrition and the Vegetarian Diet

Cutting meat and animal products out of the diet does not eliminate sugar or the many processed foods that are calorie-dense and nutrient-poor, which may be where your child is taking in extra calories. The American Dietetic Association has created a vegetarian food pyramid for lacto-ovo vegetarians, or those vegetarians who consume animal products such as milk and eggs, to help guide nutritional choices. It prescribes a daily diet of the following:

- Spare use of fats, oils, and sweets
- 0–3 servings of milk, cheese, or yogurt (with other calcium-rich substitutions for vegan children)
- 2–3 servings of dry beans, nuts, seeds, eggs, and meat substitutes such as tofu
- 3–5 servings of vegetables
- 2–4 servings of fruit
- 6–11 servings of bread, cereal, rice, and pasta

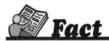 ***Fact***

Vitamins and minerals from natural food sources are more readily absorbed by the body than those contained in over-the-counter dietary supplements. If your child's vegetarian diet is balanced, vitamin supplements are usually not needed. However, you should consult with your child's pediatrician about her particular needs.

Pay particular attention to the top and the bottom of the pyramid. Sweets and fats should be minimal. (Having no animal fat in your diet to begin with will certainly help on that count.) And choosing whole-grain products for the base of the pyramid, such as whole-wheat breads and pastas and oatmeal and bran cereals, will increase dietary fiber intake.

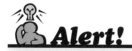
Alert!

Red meat is a major source of dietary iron, and vegetarian children can be at risk for iron-deficient anemia if they don't get enough supplementary iron in their diet. Make sure your growing child is getting enough by adding one or more of these iron-rich foods to his diet: bran flakes, sea vegetables, garbanzo beans, soybeans, spinach, tofu, pumpkin seeds, blackstrap molasses, cream of wheat, or instant oatmeal.

For Vegan Families

Children who do not consume eggs, milk, dairy, or other animal-derived products need alternative sources of vitamin B_{12}, vitamin D, and calcium in their diet. (See Chapter 6 for recommended daily allowances of vitamins and minerals.) Regular exposure to sunlight (up to fifteen minutes daily; people with darker skin tones may require slightly longer), which promotes synthesis of vitamin D by the skin, can usually provide sufficient vitamin D, but during the winter months extra dietary sources may be required. Fortified soymilk and breakfast cereal can provide adequate amounts of both B_{12} and D.

Some good sources of calcium include soy foods, many bean varieties (such as navy and great northern), dried figs, greens (collard, turnip, mustard), almonds, and broccoli. Be sure to check the labels of packaged products, particularly fortified cereals, for nutritional information.

Living with Food Allergies

According to the National Institute of Allergies and Infectious Diseases (NIAID), 3 percent of U.S. children have some form of food allergy. The percentage is higher (6 percent) for those children age three or younger; in about half of children with food allergies, they resolve by age three. The most common food allergies in children are to eggs, peanuts, and milk. Other common food allergens include tree nuts (such as walnuts), soy, shellfish, fish, and wheat. When a child with food allergies is also overweight, it may be more challenging to alter what and how much he's eating. In some cases, particularly when a child has multiple food allergies and significant dietary restrictions, it's not hard for parents to get into the habit of letting him splurge on those foods he can have, which can result in eventual weight gain.

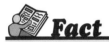 **Fact**

Linolenic and alpha-linolenic acid are two essential fatty acids found in fish and eggs that convert to the omega-3 fats. These two fatty acids are associated with heart health and protect against high triglyceride levels. Vegetarian and vegan children require a good alternate source of linolenic acid, which can be found in flaxseed, flaxseed oil, walnuts, walnut oil, canola oil, and soybean oil.

On a positive note, if your child has food allergies, you are already used to being vigilant about checking labels and asking questions in restaurants about how dishes are prepared. These good habits will work to your advantage in helping your child improve his daily diet.

Working towards weight loss or maintenance when your child has food allergies is not a simple or easy process. Adding new foods, and new foods she likes at that, has to be done with the utmost care, yet expanding her options is often the key to preventing overload on those not-so-healthy foods she currently eats too much of. If your child isn't very active, focusing on increasing exercise first may be a good strategy while you work out food options with your health-care team.

As you change your dietary patterns, you may be introducing new foods into your child's diet. Be aware that on nutritional labels, many food allergens are listed by different names which may not be obvious. For instance, "natural and/or artificial flavoring" on the ingredient list could indicate the presence of tree nut flavoring. A registered dietitian can help you learn the lingo of labels and build a dietary plan that will promote weight loss or maintenance for your child without endangering her health.

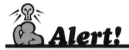

Alert!

While Americans don't consume soy by itself in large quantities, soy and soybean derivatives are used as ingredients in an overwhelming number of baked goods, sauces, soups, chips, and more. Because it is such a common prepared-food additive, eliminating it can significantly alter the nutritional balance of a child's diet if special care is not taken. If your child has a soy allergy and you haven't done so already, consult with a registered dietitian to find out how to keep his meals balanced while avoiding soy.

Picky Eaters

Your child can eat macaroni and cheese morning, noon, and night, and his total dining repertoire consists of about six foods. He refuses to consume any food or beverage that is the color green. You can't let his corn touch his chicken on the plate or both will end up in the trash.

If any of these food idiosyncrasies sounds familiar, you aren't alone. Virtually all kids have some quirks when it comes to what they'll eat and what they won't, especially the younger ones. Yet some are more particular about their meals than others. If you have a so-called picky eater on your hands, it can be easy for mealtimes to become a power struggle over what and how much your child eats.

The best way to avoid ending up with a picky eater is to introduce your child to a wide variety of healthy foods when she's just starting solids. Kids like what they know—it's safe and comfortable for them. If they're familiar with healthy foods from an early age, they'll be more likely to eat them. But if you've missed the boat on that already, there's still hope. Here are some tips that can help a fussy kid expand her culinary horizons:

- **Try, try again.** If your son turns his nose up at a new dish the first time out, don't give up just yet. New tastes and textures can sometimes overwhelm kids. Wait a few weeks, and introduce the food again. It may take five or even ten appearances before your child warms up to it. (Or he may never, but it's worth the effort to try.)
- **Make it to order.** Many kids who love raw carrots won't touch them cooked, and vice versa. When your child says he doesn't like a new food, try baking, broiling, steaming, sautéing, or stir-frying it next time to see if that flies.
- **Have a hidden agenda.** It may seem a little underhanded, but if you can sneak some spinach into a salad or bulk up your child's yogurt with a spoonful of swirled-in wheat germ, do it. Soups provide a perfect place to slide some contraband cuisine like veggies and grains past your picky eater, as do casseroles.
- **Watch your mouth.** Kids who are picky eaters often have parents who are just as picky. Don't project your own food dislikes onto your child.
- **Don't label.** Don't call your kid a picky eater—it just gives him more reason to continue being one. Along those same lines, if your child makes a special request for something new at a restaurant or in the grocery store, don't say, "I don't think you're going to like that," or he definitely won't.

Patience is the name of the game when dealing with finicky kids, so don't give up your game plan prematurely. Stay consistent, be positive, and remember that it may take a few weeks, or a few months, before your child takes the plunge and tries some new things.

 Essential

Taste isn't the only thing that turns kids off to food. If it looks or smells different than what they're used to, they may say "No thanks" before it even crosses their lips. Instituting the one-bite rule at your dinner table can help you avoid many food power struggles. Let your children know that they need to try at least one bite of a new food before deciding they don't like it. Your part of the deal is that you won't make a big issue out of it if they don't.

Letting Your Child Make Choices

Learning how to make educated decisions about snacks and meals will take some practice, even for the grown-ups in the family. Still, it's important that you share some of the decision-making responsibilities with your child so that she can gain both greater independence and a sense of self-esteem. Even though it may drive you mad to hear her ask for the same thing over and over again, it's important for her to know that her opinion counts.

Giving your child her say can also eliminate a lot of frustration about picked-over meals and wasted food. You may want to avoid asking open-ended questions like "What do you want for lunch?" The options are too numerous. For younger kids, offer two or three choices that your child can make a selection from. Older children will be fixing their own meals and snacks many times, so make sure there are plenty of healthy options available that they like.

Setting Limits

You want to keep your efforts low-key when it comes to reforming your picky eater. Standoffs at the dinner table are unproductive, anxiety-producing, and they often do nothing more than make your child dig his heels in even further. Don't insist your child clean his plate, and don't use dessert as a bargaining token. Keep using the strategies discussed in this chapter and throughout this book to hit on new food combinations and preparation methods your child enjoys. Remember to be consistent about keeping junk food out of the house.

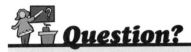 ***Question?***

Should I worry about malnutrition if my son doesn't even come close to finishing all the healthy foods I make?

Remember that a child-sized portion is only one-quarter to two-thirds of an adult portion, depending on your son's age. If you're giving him a Dad-sized portion, that could be the problem. If portions are appropriate, then perhaps he's filling up on between meal drinks and snacks. Either way, if you're offering a variety of nutritious foods, there's little need to worry about malnutrition. Remember food quality, not quantity, and don't forget the importance of an active lifestyle for your child.

At the same time, don't let your child take command of the kitchen and disrupt the family meal. There's no reason to get into the habit of cooking completely separate meals for her. Make sure there's at least one food on the table that your child enjoys with every meal. If she doesn't want to try what's served, keep a variety of easily prepared foods on hand, like whole-grain cereal, peanut butter, hard-boiled eggs, or cleaned and cut veggies, that she can eat if she wants, with the stipulation that she must prepare them herself (if of an appropriate age to do so). Tell her what's being served five minutes before the family sits down so she isn't running around the kitchen while everyone else is eating.

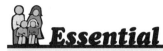 **Essential**

> It can be frustrating when you've spent a lot of time preparing something new and your child won't even try it or pushes it away after one bite. Just try not to make a big deal out of it. A good way to increase the chances of his enjoying your new creation is to let him be involved in making the meal, from grocery shopping to mixing and cooking. If he has a green thumb, he can even grow some of the ingredients with you!

Healthy Weight Loss on a Shoestring Budget

Depending on where you live, the time of year it is, and market conditions, the essential staples of a healthy diet can sometimes get pricey. But that doesn't mean you have to bypass the fresh fruits for cans of sugary fruit cocktail or skimp on other essentials. Beyond obvious strategies like buying generic when possible and using manufacturer and store coupons, there are ways to eat healthy on the cheap.

Frugal Food Choices

When buying fruits and vegetables, take advantage of seasonal farmers' markets and roadside produce stands if you have them in your area. You can usually get a much better price on produce that is direct from the source than you can on the supermarket variety, where you're also paying for shipping, advertising, and overhead. Canning, freezing, and dehydrating fruits and veggies can also help you extend your summer purchases.

If you have access to a warehouse or wholesale type of store where bulk goods and economy or restaurant-sized food staples are sold, you may be able to save some money that way. Make sure the packaging is such that you won't end up wasting half of a jumbo package of yogurt or cereal because it spoils or gets soggy. Proper airtight storage and/or freezing can help with some food products.

Seek Out the Sales

Keep an eye on store sales each week, and stock up on the better deals for later use whenever possible. For example, you may find great deals on turkey just before Thanksgiving and Christmas, so buy extra and freeze. But don't be lured into buying junk food just because it's two-for-one this week. For perishable goods, check expiration dates— a good price isn't worth much if the food will go bad in a few days.

The Real Cost of "Convenience" Foods

Another way to cut your grocery expenses is to think twice about buying heavily packaged or prepared foods. Buying precut and pre-washed produce or cereals and crackers that are divvied up into individual serving-size packages is more expensive than buying the regular stuff. The same goes for meat and poultry. It's typically much cheaper to bypass the preformed patties and seasoned and sliced strips and do the prep work yourself from less expensive cuts of meat. If you can make the time to buy whole foods and clean, slice, and repackage them yourself where necessary, your wallet will be in much better shape.

That's not to say that some of these products don't have their time and place occasionally. Time is money, and you may find that buying a bagged salad once in a while when you're strapped for time allows you to provide a more balanced meal for your family than you'd be able to prepare otherwise.

Cultural Considerations

Food can play a big part in religious and ethnic heritage, not just on special holidays and occasions but year round. Sometimes those traditions aren't so healthy. For example, many Mexican dishes call for a hefty helping of artery-clogging lard, as do a number of traditional Southern recipes.

That doesn't mean you have to say goodbye forever to refried beans or biscuits and gravy. With some imagination and perseverance, your family's old favorites can be adjusted to improve their nutritional profile. Check your local library or bookstore for one of the many health-focused cookbooks for regional and ethnic cuisines. If you can't find a near match for your particular recipe, see what substitutions are being made on the whole (such as cutting lard in favor of healthier fats, or baking instead of frying) and incorporate those ideas on your own. It may take some experimentation and a few false starts, but with some effort you'll be able to start a new food tradition.

Chronic Diseases/Disorders and Weight Loss

Living with a chronic illness is difficult enough, but when your child's condition or its associated treatment causes side effects like weight gain or restrictions in physical activity, her fitness level can deteriorate and leave her with an even more difficult battle ahead.

Is the Treatment the Trouble?

If your child is chronically ill and putting on too many pounds, the first step is determining what's behind the weight gain. Treatment of your child's illness may be the cause of the weight issue itself. For example, some children with Type 1 diabetes will initially gain weight when starting on insulin. They may shy away from exercise because of fears of low blood sugar (hypoglycemia) episodes, which could worsen the problem. Steroid treatments for asthma or lupus may cause fluid retention and subsequent weight gain. Other medications may promote weight gain through their pharmacological effects on appetite, hormones, and/or metabolism. For example, certain antidepressants can increase appetite, and the atypical antipsychotics used in the treatment of bipolar disorder are known culprits in weight gain.

Illness and Exercise

Chronic medical conditions may limit the type or amount of exercise your child gets, and this can also play a factor in weight problems. Kids who have musculoskeletal conditions like juvenile rheumatoid arthritis may find movement initially difficult, and since muscle burns more calories than fat, their low muscle tone may mean that they are burning less energy on a daily basis. Even a broken leg can be a trigger for weight gain if it sidelines your child from sufficient activity for long enough.

Appropriately treating the illness or medical condition is the first priority. That doesn't mean your child is stuck with the problem. Sometimes weight gain is just temporary. In other instances, medications or treatment regimens can be adjusted to slow or stop the mechanism behind the gain. If your child appears to be gaining weight due to a medical condition, discuss the situation with his doctor. Find out if there's a specific reason for it and if treatment adjustments are in order.

A Vicious Circle

Excess weight has been linked to many health conditions, including heart disease, high blood pressure, asthma, and joint problems (as described in Chapter 1). If your child has developed any of these conditions, weight loss may actually improve the health problems that are holding him back. It's easy to feel as if your child is stuck in a Catch-22 situation when he can't exercise due to pain or lack of stamina from a weight-related health problem, yet not exercising is contributing to his condition. In these cases it's absolutely imperative that your child have a medically guided weight-loss and fitness program supervised by his primary health-care provider. A team of pediatric health-care professionals, including an exercise physiologist or physical therapist and a registered dietitian, can put him on a safe program that can control both his weight and his health problems.

APPENDIX A

Food and Exercise
Journal Worksheets

T rack your family's progress on these fitness journal worksheets, or use the ideas here to make your own. See Chapter 5 for more information on fitness journals.

Food Diary

Sunday	
Meal/Snack	
When	
What	
How Much	
Where and Who	
What I'm Feeling	
Total Calories (optional)	
Diary:	

Monday	
Meal/Snack	
When	
What	
How Much	
Where and Who	
What I'm Feeling	
Total Calories (optional)	
Diary:	

Tuesday

Meal/Snack

When

What

How Much

Where and Who

What I'm Feeling

Total Calories (optional)

Diary:

Wednesday

Meal/Snack

When

What

How Much

Where and Who

What I'm Feeling

Total Calories (optional)

Diary:

Thursday

Meal/Snack

When

What

How Much

Where and Who

What I'm Feeling

Total Calories (optional)

Diary:

Friday

Meal/Snack

When

What

How Much

Where and Who

What I'm Feeling

Total Calories (optional)

Diary:

Saturday	
Meal/Snack	
When	
What	
How Much	
Where and Who	
What I'm Feeling	
Total Calories (optional)	
Diary:	

Activity Journal

Sunday	
Activity	Down Time
How Long	How Long
Where and Who	Where and Who
Mood	Mood
Calories Burned (optional)	
Diary:	

Monday

Activity	**Down Time**
How Long	**How Long**
Where and Who	**Where and Who**
Mood	**Mood**
Calories Burned (optional)	

Diary:

_____

_____

_____

_____

_____

_____

Tuesday

Activity	**Down Time**
How Long	**How Long**
Where and Who	**Where and Who**
Mood	**Mood**
Calories Burned (optional)	

Diary:

_____

_____

_____

_____

_____

_____

Wednesday

Activity	**Down Time**
How Long	**How Long**
Where and Who	**Where and Who**
Mood	**Mood**
Calories Burned (optional)	

Diary:

Thursday

Activity	**Down Time**
How Long	**How Long**
Where and Who	**Where and Who**
Mood	**Mood**
Calories Burned (optional)	

Diary:

Friday

Activity	**Down Time**
How Long	**How Long**
Where and Who	**Where and Who**
Mood	**Mood**
Calories Burned (optional)	

Diary:

_____

_____

_____

_____

_____

_____

_____

Saturday

Activity	**Down Time**
How Long	**How Long**
Where and Who	**Where and Who**
Mood	**Mood**
Calories Burned (optional)	

Diary:

_____

_____

_____

_____

_____

_____

_____

Online Resources

Find more information on family fitness through these education, information, advocacy, and shopping sites. Listings include parenting sites for supporting your overweight child along with teen and kid-focused fitness sites.

Kid-Focused Fitness Resources

BAM!
Body and Mind, from
the U.S. CDC
✍*www.bam.gov*

KidNetic
From the International Food
Information Council Foundation
✍*www.kidnetic.org*

**KidsHealth from the
Nemours Foundation**
For Kids and Teens
✍*www.kidshealth.org*

Parenting Support and Resources

**About Parenting of
Babies and Toddlers**
With Stephanie Brown
✍*babyparenting.about.com*

About Parenting of K-6 Children
With Kimberly Keith
✍*childparenting.about.com*

About Parenting Teens
With Denise Wittmer
✍*parentingteens.about.com*

Keep Kids Healthy
With Vincent Iannelli, MD, FAAP
✍*www.keepkidshealthy.com*

Find a Health-Care Professional

The American Academy of Pediatrics

✉141 Northwest Point Boulevard
Elk Grove Village, IL 60007-1098
✆(847) 434-4000
✆(847) 434-8000 (Fax)
✐*www.aap.org*

The American Dietetic Association

Registered Dietitian Referrals
✐*www.eatright.org*
(800) 366-1655

Find a Weight Loss or Fitness Camps

American Camping Association

✉5000 State Road 67 North
Martinsville, IN 46151
(765) 342-8456
✐*www.acacamps.org*

Child Weight-Control Programs

Shapedown

✉1323 San Anselmo Avenue
San Anselmo, CA 94960
✐*www.shapedown.com*
✆(415) 453-8886

Exercise and Physical Education

About Exercise

With Personal Trainer
Paige Waehner
✐*exercise.about.com*

American Alliance for Health, Physical Education, Recreation, and Dance

✉1900 Association Dr.
Reston, VA 20191-1598
✆(800) 213-7193
✐*www.aahperd.org*

National Center on Physical Activity and Disability

✉1640 W. Roosevelt Rd.
Chicago, IL 60608
✆(800) 900-8086
(Voice and TTY)
✐*www.ncpad.org*

The President's Council on Physical Fitness and Sports

✉Department W
200 Independence Ave., SW
Room 738-H
Washington, D.C. 20201-0004
✆(202) 690-9000
✐*www.fitness.gov*

Making Changes in the Schools

United States Department of Agriculture

Food and Nutrition Service
School Meals Program
✉3101 Park Center
Drive, Room 926
Alexandria, Virginia 22302
✍*www.fns.usda.gov*

United States Department of Education

✉400 Maryland Avenue, SW
Washington, DC 20202
✆1-800-USA-LEARN
(1-800-872-5327)
✍*www.ed.gov*

Media Literacy and Body Image

The Center for Media Literacy

✉3101 Ocean Park
Boulevard, #200
Santa Monica, CA 90405
✆310-581-0260
✍*www.medialit.org*

Just Think

✉39 Mesa St.
Suite 106
San Francisco, CA 94129
✆(415) 561-2900
✍*www.justthink.org*

Media Education Foundation

✉60 Masonic Street
Northampton, MA 01060
✆(800) 897-0089
✍*www.mediaed.org*

Media Matters

Media Education Campaign
from the American
Academy of Pediatrics
✍*www.aap.org/advocacy/
mediamatters.htm*
mediamatters@aap.org

Teen Health and the Media
Teen Futures Media Network
University of Washington
Experimental Education Unit
✉Box 357925
Seattle, WA 98195
✆(888)TEEN-NET
(888-833-6638)
✑*http://depts.washington.
edu/thmedia*

Policy and Advocacy

American Obesity Association
✉1250 24th Street, NW
Suite 300
Washington, D.C. 20037
✆(202) 776-7711
✑*www.obesity.org*

**American Public Health
Association**
✉800 I Street, NW
Washington, D.C. 20001
✆(202) 777-2742
✑*www.apha.org*

Children's Obesity Action
Children's Hospital and
Regional Medical Center
✉P.O. Box 50020/3E-2
Seattle, WA 98145
✆(206) 987-2626
✑*www.childrens
obesityaction.org*

Sleep and Your Child

**American Sleep Apnea
Association**
✉1424 K Street NW
Suite 302
Washington, D.C. 20005
✆(202) 293-3650
✑*www.sleepapnea.org*

National Sleep Foundation
✉1522 K Street, NW, Suite 500
Washington, D.C. 20005
✆(202) 347-3471
✑*www.sleepfoundation.org*

Bariatric Surgery

**American Society for
Bariatric Surgery**
✉7328 West University
Avenue, Suite F
Gainesville, FL 32607
✆(352) 331-4900
✑*www.asbs.org*

**Cincinnati Children's
Hospital Medical Center**
Comprehensive Weight
Management Center
Bariatric Surgery Program
✉3333 Burnet Avenue
Cincinnati, Ohio 45229-3039
✆(800) 344-2462
✑*www.cincinnatichildrens.org*

Clothing for Overweight Kids and Teens

Jeeny Beans
Online for girls
✎*www.jeenybeans.com*

Hey Mom, It Fits!
Online for boys and girls
✎*www.heymomitfits.com*

JC Penney's
Online and brick-and-mortar retailer offers "girls plus" and "husky boys" sizes.
✎*www.jcpenney.com*

Torrid
Online and brick-and-mortar retailer for teens and young adult women.
✎*www.torrid.com*

Vegetarian Nutrition and Lifestyle

Vegetarian Baby and Child
✉P.O. Box 388
Trenton, TX 75490
✎*www.vegetarianbaby.com*

The Vegetarian Resource Group (VRG)
✉P.O. Box 1463, Dept. IN
Baltimore, MD 21203
✆(410) 366-VEGE
✎*www.vrg.org*

Appendix C
BMI Charts

F ind your child's height in the left-hand column, then move across the row to a weight that is closest to her current weight (pounds are rounded up). The number at the top of that column is your child's BMI. For example, a child who is 50 inches tall and weighs 106 pounds has a BMI of 30.

Find Your Child's Body Mass Index (BMI)

BMI	13	14	15	16	17	18	19	20	21	22	23	24	25	26	27	28	29	30	31	32	33
Height (inches)								Weight (pounds)													
33	20	21	23	24	26	27	29	30	32	34	35	37	38	40	41	43	44	46	48	49	51
34	21	23	24	26	27	29	31	32	34	36	37	39	41	42	44	46	47	49	50	52	54
35	22	24	26	27	29	31	33	34	36	38	40	41	43	45	47	48	50	52	54	55	57
36	23	25	27	29	31	33	35	36	38	40	42	44	46	47	49	51	53	55	57	58	60
37	25	27	29	31	33	35	37	38	40	42	44	46	48	50	52	54	56	58	60	62	64
38	26	28	30	32	34	36	39	41	43	45	47	49	51	53	55	57	59	61	63	65	67
39	28	30	32	34	36	38	41	43	45	47	49	51	54	56	58	60	62	64	67	69	71
40	29	31	34	36	38	40	43	45	47	50	52	54	56	59	61	63	66	68	70	72	75
41	31	33	35	38	40	43	45	47	50	52	54	57	59	62	64	66	69	71	74	76	78
42	32	35	37	40	42	45	47	50	52	55	57	60	62	65	67	70	72	75	77	80	82
43	34	36	39	42	44	47	49	52	55	57	60	63	65	68	71	73	76	78	81	84	86
44	35	38	41	44	46	49	52	55	57	60	63	66	68	71	74	77	79	82	85	88	90
45	37	40	43	46	48	51	54	57	60	63	66	69	72	74	77	80	83	86	89	92	95
46	39	42	45	48	51	54	57	60	63	66	69	72	75	78	81	84	87	90	93	96	99
47	40	43	47	50	53	56	59	62	65	69	72	75	78	81	84	87	91	94	97	100	103
48	42	45	49	52	55	58	62	65	68	72	75	78	81	85	88	91	95	98	101	104	108

Find Your Child's Body Mass Index (BMI)

Weight (pounds)

BMI	13	14	15	16	17	18	19	20	21	22	23	24	25	26	27	28	29	30	31	32	33
Height (inches)																					
49	44	47	51	54	58	61	64	68	71	75	78	81	85	88	92	95	99	102	105	109	112
50	46	49	53	56	60	64	67	71	74	78	81	85	88	92	96	99	103	106	110	113	117
51	48	51	55	59	62	66	70	73	77	81	85	88	92	96	99	103	107	110	114	118	122
52	50	53	57	61	65	69	73	76	80	84	88	92	96	100	103	107	111	115	119	123	126
53	51	55	59	63	67	71	75	79	83	87	91	95	99	103	107	111	115	119	123	127	131
54	53	58	62	66	70	74	78	82	87	91	95	99	103	107	111	116	120	124	128	132	136
55	55	60	64	68	73	77	81	86	90	94	98	103	107	111	116	120	124	129	133	137	141
56	57	62	66	71	75	80	84	89	93	98	102	107	111	115	120	124	129	133	138	142	147
57	60	64	69	73	78	83	87	92	97	101	106	110	115	120	124	129	134	138	143	147	152
58	62	66	71	76	81	86	90	95	100	105	110	114	119	124	129	133	138	143	148	153	157
59	64	69	74	79	84	89	94	99	103	108	113	118	123	128	133	138	143	148	153	158	163
60	66	71	76	81	87	92	97	102	107	112	117	122	128	133	138	143	148	153	158	163	168
61	68	74	79	84	89	95	100	105	111	116	121	127	132	137	142	148	153	158	164	169	174
62	71	76	82	87	92	98	103	109	114	120	125	131	136	142	147	153	158	164	169	175	180
63	73	79	84	90	95	101	107	112	118	124	129	135	141	146	152	158	163	169	174	180	186
64	75	81	87	93	99	104	110	116	122	128	134	139	145	151	157	163	168	174	180	186	192

Find Your Child's Body Mass Index (BMI)

BMI Height (inches)	13	14	15	16	17	18	19	20	21	22	23	24	25	26	27	28	29	30	31	32	33
									Weight (pounds)												
65	78	84	90	96	102	108	114	120	126	132	138	144	150	156	162	168	174	180	186	192	198
66	80	86	92	99	105	111	117	123	130	136	142	148	154	161	167	173	179	185	192	198	204
67	83	89	95	102	108	114	121	127	134	140	146	153	159	166	172	178	185	191	197	204	210
68	85	92	98	105	111	118	124	131	138	144	151	157	164	171	177	184	190	197	203	210	217
69	88	94	101	108	115	121	128	135	142	148	155	162	169	176	182	189	196	203	209	216	223
70	90	97	104	111	118	125	132	139	146	153	160	167	174	181	188	195	202	209	216	223	230
71	93	100	107	114	121	129	136	143	150	157	164	172	179	186	193	200	207	215	222	229	236
72	95	103	110	117	125	132	140	147	154	162	169	176	184	191	199	206	213	221	228	235	243
73	98	106	113	121	128	136	144	151	159	166	174	181	189	197	204	212	219	227	234	242	250
74	101	109	116	124	132	140	148	155	163	171	179	186	194	202	210	218	225	233	241	249	257
75	104	112	120	128	136	144	152	160	168	176	184	192	200	208	216	224	232	240	248	256	264
76	106	115	123	131	139	147	156	164	172	180	188	197	205	213	221	230	238	246	254	262	271
77	109	118	126	134	143	151	160	168	177	185	193	202	210	219	227	236	244	253	261	269	278
78	112	121	129	138	147	155	164	173	181	190	199	207	216	225	233	242	250	259	268	276	285

CDC Growth Charts: United States

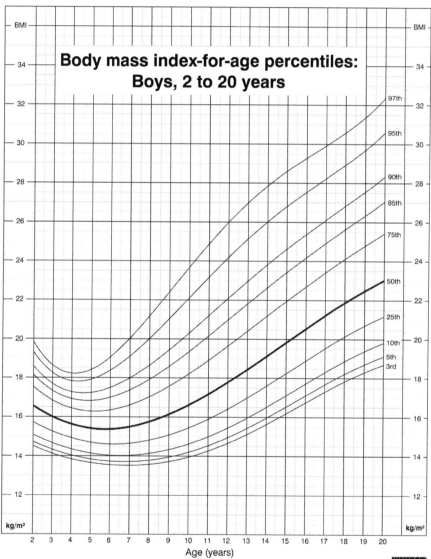

Body mass index-for-age percentiles: Boys, 2 to 20 years

BMI

97th
95th
90th
85th
75th
50th
25th
10th
5th
3rd

Age (years)

kg/m²

Published May 30, 2000.
SOURCE: Developed by the National Center for Health Statistics in collaboration with the National Center for Chronic Disease Prevention and Health Promotion (2000).

SAFER·HEALTHIER·PEOPLE™

CDC Growth Charts: United States

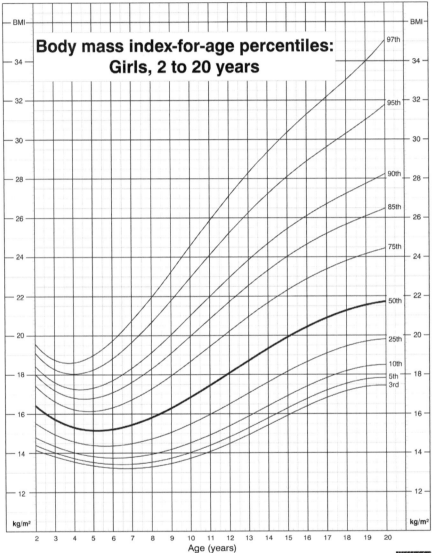

Body mass index-for-age percentiles: Girls, 2 to 20 years

BMI

34

32

30

28

26

24

22

20

18

16

14

12

kg/m²

97th
95th
90th
85th
75th
50th
25th
10th
5th
3rd

Age (years)

2 3 4 5 6 7 8 9 10 11 12 13 14 15 16 17 18 19 20

Published May 30, 2000.
SOURCE: Developed by the National Center for Health Statistics in collaboration with the National Center for Chronic Disease Prevention and Health Promotion (2000).

SAFER·HEALTHIER·PEOPLE™

Index

A

Acknowledging problem, 33–35
Acronyms (on labels), 75–76
Activity. *See* Exercise/activity
Advertising, 16–17, 247–48
Aerobic training, 132, 151–52
Age, weight and, 231–53. *See also*
  Teens
  adult issues, 12–13, 251–53
  baby fat and, 231–32
  hearing hunger, 233
  infants, 231–33
  peer influence and, 238–39
  puberty, 5, 241–42
  school-aged to preteens, 237–38
  teens, 241–51
  toddlers/preschool, 234–37
Anger, 38–39
Atkins diet, 97

B

Babies. *See* Age, weight and
Binge-eating disorder (BED), 25, 164–
  66, 224. *See also* Slipups
Blame, 34
BMI. *See* Body mass index (BMI)
Body image, 161–62
Body mass index (BMI), 3–4, 30–32,
  232, 293–98
Body shapes, 232
Boredom, 230
Breastfeeding, 27, 107–8
Budget-conscious weight loss, 275–76
Bullying. *See* Teasing

C

Calories
  burn rates, 143–44, 152
  daily requirements, 58–59
  3500-calorie equation, 59–60

Carbohydrates/fiber, 77–79, 95–99. *See*
  also Sugar consumption
Causes, of weight problems, 6–10
Charting growth, 28–33, 293–98
Cholesterol, 79–81, 114–15, 267
Clean plate syndrome, 90–91
College, 252
Communicating
  with children, 34–35, 37–40
  with doctor, 35–36
Counseling. *See* Support
Cultural considerations, 2, 276–77
Cybersloths, 7–8

D

Dating, 243–44
Depression, 122–23, 174–77
Diabetes, 4, 211, 277
Diet. *See also* Eating appropriately;
    Eating inappropriately; Food; Food
    labels
  exercise and. *See* Exercise/activity
  lifestyle change vs., 40
  sibling relationships and, 51–53, 236
Diets, 93–105. *See also specific diet*
    names; Weight loss
  balance and, 94–95
  franchise organizations, 100–102
  infants/toddlers and, 233
  low-carb, 95–99
  low-fat, 99–100
  negative connotations, 93–94
  nutritional counseling, 102–4
  short- vs. long-term fixes, 105
Doctor
  assessments by, 32–33. *See also*
      Body mass index (BMI)
  talking with, 35–36
  weight loss and, 64–65
Drug therapy, 249

THE *EVERYTHING®*
PARENT'S GUIDES SERIES

Expert Advice for Parents in Need of Answers

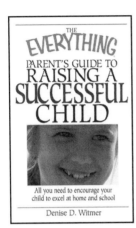

THE
EVERYTHING
PARENT'S GUIDE TO
RAISING A
SUCCESSFUL
CHILD

All you need to encourage your
child to excel at home and school

Denise D. Witmer

ISBN: 1-59337-043-1

How do I make sure my child is successful? What defines a successful child? Is my child already "successful"?

As parents struggle with these questions on a daily basis, *The Everything® Parent's Guide to Raising a Successful Child* helps put their fears to rest, providing them with professional, reassuring advice on how to raise a "successful" child according to their own standards.

This title walks parents through all emotional, intellectual, and physical aspects of development, including: building character, choosing—and limiting—extracurricular activities, disciplining effectively, ensuring a quality education, and instilling morals and values.

For parents of children with autism, daily activities such as grocery shopping or getting dressed can become extremely challenging. *The Everything® Parent's Guide to Children with Autism* offers practical advice, gentle reassurance, and real-life scenarios to help your family get through each day. Written by Adelle Jameson Tilton, the About.com Guide to Autism, this sensitive work helps you:

- Communicate effectively with your child
- Deal with meltdowns—public or private
- Keep your family together as one unit
- Find a school that suits your child's needs—integration vs. special education
- Learn about assistive devices, such as computers and picture boards
- Find intervention and support groups

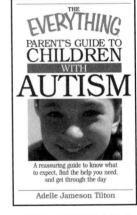

THE
EVERYTHING
PARENT'S GUIDE TO
CHILDREN
WITH
AUTISM

A reassuring guide to know what
to expect, find the help you need,
and get through the day

Adelle Jameson Tilton

ISBN: 1-59337-041-5

All titles are trade paperback, 6" x 9", $14.95

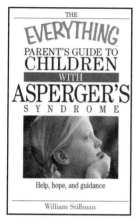

THE

EVERYTHING

PARENT'S GUIDE TO

CHILDREN

WITH

ASPERGER'S

S Y N D R O M E

Help, hope, and guidance

William Stillman

ISBN: 1-59337-153-5

While children with Asperger's are generally of average or above average intelligence, they experience challenges with social skills, communication, and coordination, among other issues.

The Everything® Parent's Guide to Children with Asperger's Syndrome is an informative resource that helps parents recognize areas in which their child needs support. Filled with helpful hints and practical guidance, this authoritative work is designed to provide parents with the latest information on the best treatments and therapies available, education options, and ways to make life easier for parent and child on a day-to-day basis.

Also including information on resources, and vetted for accuracy by Diane Twachtman-Cullen, Ph.D., this title is a must-read for parents of children affected by ASD.

The Everything® Parent's Guide to Children with Dyslexia by Abigail Marshall—manager of *www.dyslexia.com*— gives you a complete understanding of what dyslexia is, how to identify the signs, and what you can do to help your child. This authoritative book seeks to alert parents to the special needs associated with this learning disability and offers practical suggestions for getting involved in the classroom. You will learn how to:

* Select the right treatment programs for your child
* Secure an IEP
* Choose a school and reduce homework struggles
* Develop your child's skills with the use of assistive technology
* Maintain open communication and offer support

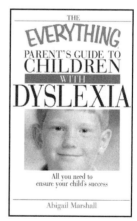

THE

EVERYTHING

PARENT'S GUIDE TO

CHILDREN

WITH

DYSLEXIA

All you need to ensure your child's success

Abigail Marshall

ISBN: 1-59337-135-7

Available wherever books are sold
Or call 1-800-872-5627 or visit us at *www.everything.com*

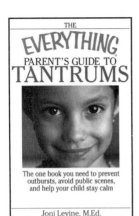

THE
EVERYTHING
PARENT'S GUIDE TO
TANTRUMS

The one book you need to prevent
outbursts, avoid public scenes,
and help your child stay calm

Joni Levine, M.Ed.

ISBN: 1-59337-321-X

A child's tantrum can happen at virtually any time—but whenever or wherever one occurs, it's always inconvenient, frustrating, and embarrassing for a parent and sometimes dangerous for the child herself. *The Everything® Parent's Guide to Tantrums* teaches parents to identify various triggers that provoke extreme reactions and helps them strategize ways to calm down their children and minimize any long-term effect.

Child care specialist Joni Levine, M.Ed., also helps parents to:
- Identify warning signs of a tantrum
- Cool off the child before the tantrum escalates
- Develop strategies and interventions to redirect the behavior
- Handle the outbursts without losing your own cool

If you're looking for the facts about how this disorder may affect your child, it's hard to know where to turn. *The Everything® Parent's Guide to Children with ADD/ADHD*, written by child psychologist Linda Sonna, gives you the clear answers and accurate information about the signs, symptoms, and treatments of this disorder that you need.

The Everything® Parent's Guide to Children with ADD/ADHD helps you:

- Learn the differences and similarities between ADD and ADHD
- Obtain and understand the diagnosis
- Weigh the pros and cons of medication
- Find the right treatment
- Discipline your child effectively

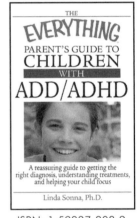

THE
EVERYTHING
PARENT'S GUIDE TO
CHILDREN
WITH
ADD/ADHD

A reassuring guide to getting the
right diagnosis, understanding treatments,
and helping your child focus

Linda Sonna, Ph.D.

ISBN: 1-59337-308-2

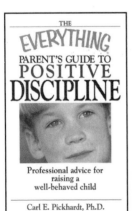

THE
EVERYTHING
PARENT'S GUIDE TO
POSITIVE
DISCIPLINE

Professional advice for
raising a
well-behaved child

Carl E. Pickhardt, Ph.D.

ISBN: 1-58062-978-4

The Everything® Parent's Guide to Positive Discipline gives you all you need to help you cope with behavior issues. Written by noted psychologist Dr. Carl E. Pickhardt, this authoritative, practical book provides you with professional advice on dealing with everything from getting your kids to do their homework to teaching them to respect their elders. This title also shows parents how to:

- Set priorities
- Promote communication
- Establish the connection between choice and consequence
- Enforce punishment
- Change discipline style to reflect the age of the child
- Work with your partner as a team